LUCKY TO BE ALIVE

MY REMARKABLE RECOVERY FROM SUICIDAL MADNESS

THOMAS RICKE

ILLUMIFY MEDIA GLOBAL
Littleton, Colorado

CONTENTS

Chapter 1

I can't remember who started singing that night forty-five years ago. It could have been one of the college professors or one of the factory workers or even one of the prostitutes. We were all jammed into the back of a paddy wagon with a screaming siren and flashing red lights that bounced off the buildings we passed on the empty early morning streets. We had been drinking and playing poker in an illegal after-hours place in the deep Detroit inner city. Tange's opened at 2 a.m. after the legal bars closed.

I was a reporter for the *Detroit Free Press* at the time, and the illegal basement called Tange's was one of my favorite places. I would go there when my drinking could not put out the fire in my head that would keep me awake for days and nights.

"America, America, God shed his grace on thee," we sang.

"Shut up back there for Christ's sake," the cop in the passenger seat screamed at us as he banged his nightstick on the front of our cage.

But we didn't stop, not until we pulled into police head-quarters.

We were arrested in what was commonly called a "blind pig," and after we were processed and fingerprinted we would have to wait in a cold cement cell until court opened later that morning.

During the summer of 1967 a paddy wagon (could it have been the same one we used that morning?) pulled up to a blind pig on Twelfth Street. In a raid just like the one that caught us, police led customers from an upstairs apartment onto the street and into the wagon. An indignant crowd gathered and pelted the police with rocks and bottles.

Bricks and bottles and soon fires and looting—the Detroit riots of 1967 started when a group the same size as ours climbed into the back of a paddy wagon.

Forty-three people lost their lives the week of that riot, and the staff of the *Detroit Free Press* won a Pulitzer Prize for its coverage of the week-long bloody battle.

I had brought a friend with me to Tange's that morning. She was a reporter for the *Detroit News*, our competing paper, and she wanted to see for herself what Tange's was like. I lost her after we climbed out of the paddy wagon when they guided the men and women into two separate groups. The women got nicer cells. The men were crowded into one large concrete cell with a wooden bench against a wall that could hold only a few of them. Those of us who had to stand watched the sunrise through the bars of the cell's only window. The expressways were filling up with cars driven by white people who were driving on the congested roads from the suburbs to the city, Chevys, Chryslers, and Fords.

"Don't worry too much," the cop who was supposed to watch us said as he stood in front of the large cell, "you will be charged with a misdemeanor, loitering in a place of illegal occupation. Most of the charges get kicked out by the court. And if you are convicted, you will probably get a suspended sentence or a $25 fine at the most. We're not after you, it's the men who run these places we're after."

They marched us to another holding cell in the Frank Murphy Hall of Justice where the courts opened about 10 a.m. The court officer began to call out the names of men to go in front of the judge. They left for the courtroom two or three at a time.

About half an hour after court opened, the court officer

announced all the names of the people arrested at Tange's. We were free to go, he said. The charges had been dropped.

Tange was waiting for us in the lobby of the court building apologizing for our arrests and telling us to be sure and visit his place again.

Months later I found out what really happened. Tange was driven downtown in a police car. He lost about $800 during the ride. He was able to return to his place and reopen it before he returned to the courthouse to greet us when we were released.

Tange had competition across the street where Society Slim ran his blind pig. I visited both of them but preferred Tange's because more newspaper people went there. Tange and Society Slim used to call the police on each other hoping the police would put their competition out of business. The police weren't interested in putting either place out of business. They didn't sell dope at either place. They offered their customers liquor, gambling, and sometimes prostitutes who worked on their own. Finally, the police wouldn't make any money by closing them.

I lived a double life during my early and mid-twenties when I worked as a newspaper reporter. I was a good reporter and writer. My feature stories were often run in the *Sunday Magazine* or on the first page of the Sunday feature section. I won awards for my writing. While I was becoming a successful reporter there were times I became so depressed I called in sick and stayed in bed. I would try to feel better by drinking a lot but I found that alcohol only made the depression worse.

Other times I could be the life of the party. And when the times were good I had enhanced sensitivity. I could feel pain, sorrow, and soaring emotions from people I wrote about and write it in a way that made readers feel the same emotions.

Here is a story I reported and wrote for the *Detroit Free Press Sunday Magazine* when I was twenty-four. It is fairly representative of my work for the Detroit paper.

Chapter 2

This was the cover story of the *Detroit Free Press Sunday Magazine* was an article I wrote published on October 4, 1970:

It's 2 a.m., May 8, 1970, and the old pale green apartment building called Stonehead Manor at 4330 Lincoln near Wayne State University is quiet. Most of the building's 16 residents are asleep, planning to march later in the day in a downtown peace demonstration.

Upstairs in apartment 9 four teenagers who have just started living their own lives away from home are sleeping. Sandra Garland and Scott Kabran are together in one of two beds in the bedroom. Gregory Walls is in the other. Anthony Brown is on the living room couch.

Sandra Garland, stone-faced and soft-hearted, had left home the weekend before. She is small, short and has waist-length black hair. She holds a part-time job, is a year ahead of her age group in school and goes to church every Sunday. She also smokes dope, drops acid and digs young men.

Scott Kabran, 18, thin, frail, with shoulder-length red hair, writes poetry about women, love and death. He is an orphan whose foster mother died when he was six. His friends say he was searching for the mother's love he missed as a child. He has no brothers or sisters and is used to getting his own way.

Gregory Walls, 17, black, well-built and handsome, has the gift of touching others' lives with happiness. He is working two part-time jobs and is studying to be an actor.

He left home on his own so his mother would have one less mouth to feed. He is planning to go to Europe on a 13-week scholarship in dramatic arts.

Anthony Brown, 16, good looking and browned haired, tells friends he is 19.

He is trying to forget that his father and mother drank too much and that the whole town of Coral, Michigan knew. A runaway from a boys' training school, Tony is friendly and likes to help others clean their apartments and fix things. He is almost always stoned.

As they sleep, the song "I had a Dream" by John Sebastian, the song that opened the Woodstock Music Festival, drifts from a first floor apartment.

I had a dream last night
What a lovely dream it was
I dreamed we all were all right
Happy in the Land of Oz

A car screeches to a stop in front of 4330 Lincoln. Arville D. Garland and his wife, Martha, jump out and run to the apartment house door.

Garland, 45, six feet tall and over 200 pounds, is a railroad engineer from Tennessee who had a big American flag proudly displayed over his living room mantel. He is a member of the Detroit Police Emergency Reserves. He is Sandra's father.

Garland and his wife have been searching for Sandra for five days.

Garland kicks open the apartment house door. He has a .45 caliber Luger in one hand and a .38 caliber revolver in the other. His pockets are stuffed with bullets.

Garland and his wife run up the stairs to apartment 9.

"Sandy, Sandy," he screams. There is no answer. He puts a shoulder to the door and forces it open. Martha follows him in. They barge into a large room with posters...John Sinclair ("Revolution is poetry," it says)...W.C. Fields...a policeman with a bullet hole in his head.

Anthony Brown, sleeping on the couch, does not wake up. To his left, Garland sees a cascade of colorful beads hanging in a doorway. He pushes them aside and walks into the bedroom.

Gregory Walls is in a bed directly in front of Garland. To the left is a dartboard of Lyndon Johnson's face with several darts in Johnson's head.

To his right, naked under a sheet, are his daughter and Scott Kabran. Above the bed is a poster that reads, "Howe Military School."

Scott wakes up to see the two guns pointed at him.

Sandy wakes up too and yells, "Mama, make him stop, make him stop."

Kabran and Garland struggle. Garland's gun points toward his daughter. The shots fire.

"My baby's dead! My baby's dead! You've killed my baby," Mrs. Garland screams at her husband's side.

Garland pumps two shots in Scott Kabran's head. He turns and fires one shot into Gregory Walls' head. Garland goes into the living room and shoots Anthony Brown and yells, "Get up, boy, get up," at the dead body.

Garland reloads his guns and runs into the hallway where he meets residents of the building awakened by the shooting.

"Where's Donna? Where's Donna? If you don't tell me I'll kill you all," Garland screams. He is looking for Donna Potts, Sandra's girlfriend whom Garland blames for influencing his daughter.

Garland runs down the stairs to Donna's apartment and shoots the lock off her door. But Donna hides in the bathroom and Garland does not find her.

"No Donna," Garland tells his wife.

Mr. and Mrs. Garland walk out to their car and drive to the

Vernor police station where he tells the desk sergeant, "I have just killed my daughter and her hippie friends."

He is crying softly.

Months have passed. The four teenagers who died at the hand of the generation that brought them into this world have been buried. Arville D. Garland is in jail, racked with guilt and fear, awaiting trial.

Many people say that Sandra and Scott and Greg and Tony deserved to be punished for the way they lived. For their long hair and their unconventional life styles. For their hard rock music. For their dope. People say they might have even done what Garland did, if they walked in on their daughter naked in bed, asleep with a hippie, a black boy in another bed in the same room.

Other, younger people say they have contempt for the way Arville Garland lived. Young people sifting through the ironies of life on their own.

Young people who can't understand how their parents get drunk on alcohol yet shrink at the thought of dope; how their parents treat the American flag like a sacred tabernacle; how their parents keep telling them what a great country they live in when all they see is poverty and racism and injustice. People who say they would destroy the things Arville Garland held dear and perhaps even Arville Garland himself.

For these people who do not understand each other, we introduce Sandra and Greg and Scott and Tony and Arville D. Garland. After you know them, decide what you would have done. For they did not really know each other.

Anthony A. Brown

Whenever Tony Brown got stoned, which was often, he liked to put on a rubber gorilla mask and run up and down the stairs of Stonehead Manor yelling, "freeeaak."

He wore another invisible mask he never took off. That mask made him appear to be a worldly, yet friendly, 19-year-old. It made him just like the other residents of the building who would not have accepted him as an equal if they had known he was only 16. The girls would not have liked him as much. The guys would have talked down to him. So Tony became 19. He threw away three years of his life he never got a chance to reclaim.

Under the mask Tony was still a sensitive 16-year-old.

"Just a kid at heart, a kid looking for the love he never got at home," said a member of his family who did not want to be identified.

Tony's father was a Navy career man. He was also the town drunk. Tony's mother is now Mrs. Patricia Hart, 37 and on her third marriage.

When Tony was 12, his father came home very drunk one day and started picking on his older stepsister, Sheila, who was making dinner. Sheila was 15 and had just begun dating boys. Her stepfather asked her exactly what she was doing on her dates. They argued. Brown hit Sheila and her mother. Then he got a shotgun and kept the whole family at gunpoint until the state police came. The incident broke up the shaky marriage.

For the next two years, Tony's mother ran around a lot and drank a lot, and often brought her men friends home. In the small town of Coral, Michigan, she was talked about a lot.

Sheila ran off and got married. Tony started skipping school, because he couldn't bear knowing what his classmates were saying.

In 1968 after his mother became Mrs. Lawrence Hart, Tony ran away from home and was caught and ran away from home and was caught and ran away from home again. And was caught again. They put him in D.J. Maxey's Training School at Whitmore Lake.

Last winter Tony came back to Coral to live with the Frank Wilcox family. He and young Larry Wilcox broke into the town's barber shop one night and stole $12. They sent Tony back to Whitmore Lake.

In January there was a court hearing. Patricia Hart told the judge she didn't want Tony back because he would ruin her happy home life. Tony cried and told the judge he didn't want to go home either. He went back to Whitmore Lake.

On March 17, Tony ran away from the training school and came to Detroit.

After Tony was dead, his mother sat at a kitchen table in a farmhouse in Coral holding her new baby son and crying. She broke down and finally said, "Tony was a good boy. He never hurt anyone. He was the only one of my kids who brought home a bird with a broken wing and kept it until it healed."

Tony missed his family in Coral. Two weeks before he was killed, he borrowed money and took a bus home where his grandmother and mother gave him some clothes. He lied and told them he was doing fine in Detroit working at Hudson's.

A few days before he was killed, Tony gave a girl in the building his grandmother's phone number "just in case something happens to me."

Tony took off his 19-year-old mask one time before he died. "One night we were having a party," said Mary Ann Seggern, "and we were sitting around and Tony and I rapped for a long time. Finally he said. 'You know what's weird? I'm only sixteen and I'm living like I'm nineteen and I don't know if I like it at all.'"

"The night he was killed Tony turned us on to some good weed," Miss Seggern recalled. "He went to sleep stoned and never woke up. Tony didn't have an apartment on his own here. If he had slept on a different couch, he would still be alive."

Gregory Walls

The day before Mother's Day – the day after Greg was killed – his mother, Mrs. Annie Revel, received 12 long stemmed roses.

The card read, "To mom on Mother's Day, love Greg." Mrs. Revel, who works to provide for seven of her nine children from two marriages, gazed at the flowers lovingly.

"When he first mentioned moving out, when he was 16," she said, "I discouraged him. But when he brought it up again at 17, I felt he was old enough to know what he wanted and I gave him my blessing." She turned and said she did not want to talk anymore.

Greg worked two part-time jobs – one in the florist shop in the afternoons, the other in the grocery next to the florist shop in the evenings.

Mrs. Mary O'Neill, who worked with Greg as a clerk in the evenings, nervously lit a cigarette and tried to hold back the tears when she talked about Greg.

"We all have prejudices instilled in us," she said. "If he didn't do anything else, he taught me – his skin is black and mine is white – he taught me we're the same. I have a son his age and when Greg would tell me how he worried about his deodorant and socks and showers, just like my son tells me, well, Greg was exactly like my son in every respect.

"He had high ideals and enormous ambitions," she said. "He worked hard at school. He was so excited about going to Europe. I really loved him, I really did."

Greg attended night school at Cass Technical High School. He studied drama and was learning to write scripts for radio and television.

One night after Greg and Scott were settled in their in their new apartment on Lincoln, they borrowed some good silverware and wine glasses and cooked a roast beef dinner with all of the trimmings. They invited Greg's mother and Scott's father for the evening.

The Jewish man and the black woman both say they will always remember that night. All the residents in the building were told to keep their stereos quiet for that special evening.

"We sat and talked for hours," Stanley Kabran recalled, "it was wonderful."

Mrs. Charles Woods, who lives at 20415 Mark Twain – in Detroit's still predominately white Northwest side – lost her teenage daughter in a tragic accident at a high school rock festival about the time Greg moved away from home.

"I never heard of Greg before he came over one Sunday after my daughter died," she said. "Greg was a beautiful kid. He just came to the door with flowers and said he was a classmate of

Lynn's and was very sorry. He promised me that as long as he was alive he would visit me every Sunday."

"He sent flowers on Thanksgiving and a card at Easter and Christmas. He never missed a Sunday. He always brought different kids with him. It got so I looked forward to his visits.

"His was the hand that helped me through, the hand I held all the way… He sent me a rose tree for Mother's Day. It can be planted in the yard. Every time I look at it, I will think of him.

"I am more grieved over Greg's death than I was over my own daughter's," she said.

Scott Kabran

When Scott Kabran was a skinny little blond kid, he used to walk down the street in front of his house at 14015 Curtis and tell other children: "I'm better than you 'cause I'm adopted. You were just born, I was picked."

"He said that," Scott's father, Stanley Kabran, the owner of a northwest Detroit flower shop, explained, "because we always used to tell him that he was doubly blessed to be adopted."

When Scott was six, his foster mother died unexpectedly. "I never remarried," Kabran said, sitting in his comfortably furnished duplex. "Every time I would introduce Scott to a lady friend, he would tell me later, 'You've got to get a mommy just like my mommy.'"

Scott attended Windship Elementary School and spent the eighth, ninth and tenth grades at Howe Military School where he sang in the choir and played in the band.

When Scott was 14 he looked like a ten-year-old. An obstruction in his digestive organs prevented him from growing, but he had surgery when he was 14 and soon Scott began to grow like a weed.

Scott was quiet most of the time. His friends said he often looked depressed. When his feelings did come out, they came out on paper. He wrote poetry. He wanted to attend Oakland University and study creative writing.

"I told him he couldn't make any money writing, especially poetry," Scott's father said, "but he was determined that's what he wanted to do.

"He would see me when he worked part-time in the (florist) shop. Sometimes we would sit down and have a good cry. I left home when I was 18 too.

"He used to say, 'Dad, I don't want to cause you any aggravation. I just want to be myself.'

"You know what I miss the most?" Kabran said, "I look around and see the wind blowing and watch for his long red hair in the wind. The hair I kept bugging him to get cut. It was so beautiful blowing in the wind…"

According to his friends, Scott spent a lot more time than they did thinking about and seeing young women. They say that when Scott liked a girl, he fell in love quickly and became so possessive that he often drove the girl away.

One girl Scott loved was 18-year-old Sharon Czech.

"I met him over at the apartment," she said, "and we hit it off right away. I used to wear a sailor hat and he used to wear a cowboy hat and we would walk downtown and go window shopping.

"He had asked me to marry him and so I said yes, and we had a ceremony right in the hallway of our school (Bishop Gallagher). Greg was a minister in the Universal Life Church – that's where you send away and they make you a minister – and he married us.

"After that he introduced me to his friends as his wife. But there was always so many people coming in and out of his apartment we hardly ever kissed," she said.

Sharon's parents told her to stop seeing Scott.

Soon Donna Potts moved into a downstairs apartment in Stonehead Manor and a girl named Sandy Garland began visiting her almost every morning on her way to school. Scott noticed Sandy and started hanging out when she arrived. Soon they were taking rides in Sandy's new Volkswagen and eating breakfast together with Donna. Scott was falling in love again.

Sandra Garland

Sandy's red 1970 Volkswagen with the Wayne State University sticker in the back window is still parked in the driveway of the home where she grew up at 5755 Otis on Detroit's southwest side.

The Volkswagen was a 17th birthday present from her parents. They were proud of her, an excellent student who graduated from Chadsey High School at 16 and was taking pre-medical courses at Wayne State University just after she turned 17.

Five days before she was killed, Sandy left the Volkswagen in the driveway and loaded all of her clothes and books and even her big brown teddy bear into a friend's car.

Her moving out climaxed two years of growing tension between Sandy and her parents.

When she was a junior in high school Sandy started to wear strings of beads around her neck and her skirts became shorter. She and Donna Potts, Sandy's best friend since they were both eight years old, became what they called "freaks" together.

"There were only a few of us at school," Donna Potts said proudly. "The other kids called us hippies and freaks but we were the first ones. Now they are all into it."

Donna and Sandy started using drugs. Sandy kept marijuana and hashish in her room at home.

Sandy's mother worried constantly that her daughter was becoming a hippie. "I wanted her to grow up to be a nice young lady with high morals and dignity," she said.

Sandy was only allowed to use her new car to drive to and from work, school and church.

Mrs. Garland told her friends that Sandy had been through "every phase in the book" and considered her daughter's long-haired boyfriends and her mod clothes another phase she was anxious for her to grow out of.

Mrs. Garland did not suspect Sandy of using drugs. She asked Sandy about it once and Sandy told her, "No, Mother, not at all."

"I just would not let her run loose," Mrs. Garland told a friend. "She had to be home by midnight and nearly always was.

She always obeyed us around the house. We are just like millions of parents and Sandy was just like millions of daughters growing up."

During her last year of high school Sandy started experimenting with harder drugs.

Donna Potts recalls: "One Sunday at a rock concert at Tartar (Tartar field at Wayne State University), I took a hit and a half of brown mescaline and Sandy took one hit (tablet). I freaked out. I kept hitting everyone and tearing at people with my hands like claws and screaming. Sandy was tripped too and didn't know what to do so she drove me to her house.

"Her parents were really shocked and called my mother, who came over. They called the police and, anyway, I ended up in a straightjacket on the way to a hospital. They pumped my stomach and I spent a week there."

After that incident Mrs. Garland and Mrs. Potts told the girls they couldn't see each other. But Mr. Garland intervened and let them continue their friendship.

"Sandy really loved her father," Donna said, "And he really loved her. She ran away from home for a day last fall and when he found her and brought her back he cried and told her he would do anything to keep her at home – and the next minute he told her if she ever left again, he would chain her up."

Sandy and Donna went to church every Sunday and usually took their brothers Douglas, 14, and a baby brother, Scott.

Clifford Crosby is a 16-year-old black who dated Sandy occasionally without her parent's knowledge.

"She would really start to enjoy herself and have a good time," Crosby said, "and then she would change and say, 'I have to be home.'

"She could never really enjoy herself because she always worried about her parents finding out what she was doing.

"I remember one day when she was really happy. She and Donna just moved into their apartment and they both jumped up and down and Sandy kept saying, 'We've got our own apartment. We got our own apartment.'"

"The night she was killed," Donna said, "she and Scott talked about going to New York together. One thing though, she really loved her father. She said she had trouble with her mother, but her father was like her."

Arville D. Garland

Arville Garland's hair is mostly grey and white now. Before May 8, it was black with only traces of grey. He is living on the seventh floor of the Wayne County Jail.

Other prisoners torment him because he killed his daughter and her three friends, but he is his own worst tormenter.

Doctors who have interviewed him at the jail say he is driving himself crazy with guilt and fear about what will happen to him and the rest of his family. They say Garland is so polite and respectful to them and everyone else that he is offensive without realizing it.

He tried to escape from Ypsilanti State Hospital (where doctors found him mentally fit to stand trial) after he was told he would have to return to the jail.

Garland was born on September 21, 1924, in Erwin, Tennessee, a town of about 4,000 in the southeast corner of the state.

He went to grade school and high school there and then spent three years in the Navy.

"He wanted to be a professional football player," said Garland's father, Roy Garland, 72, "but we talked him out of it. We told him too many kids got hurt that way.

"We raised him up right. We raised him in the church. He had a good home. He never lied. If he saw money laying around he would ask who it belonged to and try to give it back to the owner."

Roy Garland retired seven years ago after working for the railroad for 45 years.

"There's never been a better boy," Roy said. "He always respected his parents and would do anything he could to help us. I was always a good Christian and Arvie, he would help some folks who are down and out, folks I wouldn't help myself."

When Arville Garland returned home from the Navy, he attended Milligan College in Milligan, Tenn., where he earned a bachelor's degree in education and a state teacher certificate. Then he attended the University of Tennessee in Knoxville to work on his master's degree. He quit after six months.

Arville Garland married Martha who grew up on a farm and never completed high school.

Years later, when her children were in Detroit schools, Mrs. Garland went back to school herself and received a high school diploma. She was attending Wayne State Community College before Sandy was killed.

Garland worked for a while in the roundhouse gang at the railroad where his father worked. "He didn't see much future in it," Roy Garland said, "so he packed up his family and moved up there to Michigan."

Garland got a job at the New York Central Railroad as an engineer. He stayed with the company when it merged with the Penn Central.

Doctors who have interviewed Garland said he told them he did not become a teacher because he was just "an average" student. He did not feel he would be a good teacher. They said he suffers from feelings of inferiority and inadequacy.

Garland devoted most of his adult life to working and providing for his family. His fellow workers said he carried a gun to work sometimes. He was quiet and kept to himself. He did not smoke and rarely drank.

He was a strong patriot, but he believed in individual rights. He told Mrs. Garland that Sandy's boyfriends had a right to have long hair. He worried about them, though, and about their influence on his daughter.

"He didn't have much in common with folks in town up there," Roy Garland said. "He told me he would rather work than just be sitting around or visiting with folks."

Garland sent his parents money regularly until he bought the

Volkswagen for Sandy. "He used up all his savings on that car," Roy said. "He loved her the best. I think he loved her too much.

"He told me has shed gallons of tears since it (the shootings) happened. He told me he blacked out after he accidentally shot Sandy. He said, 'Oh, if I would only have stopped and thought.'"

Garland missed two shifts at work the week he was looking for Sandy. After the shifts he did work, he spent most of his hours awake worrying about her.

The Tuesday before the killings Garland just missed finding Sandy, who had stopped at the apartment to visit. The caretaker, Rubin Rodriguez, showed Garland to Donna's apartment and Garland remarked, "That's Sandy's lamp. That's her dress. Where is she?"

Sandy was in an upstairs apartment at the time, but Rodriguez didn't say so.

Keith Potter, one of the residents, said, "Garland offered me $50 to tell where Sandy was." Porter told him he didn't know.

Later that day, Garland visited Donna Potts at the downtown clothing store where she works as a sales clerk. "He told me he knew I knew where Sandy was and he told me that if I didn't tell him, he would kill her," Donna said.

Rodriguez said, "He told me he was going to bring her back home, dead or alive."

Garland's version of the slayings is that when he was scuffling with Scott Kabran, his gun went off accidentally and shot his daughter in the head. He says that after that he blacked out and doesn't remember killing Greg and Scott and Tony.

His lawyers say they will defend him on the grounds that he was temporarily insane. He is charged with three counts of first-degree murder and one count of second-degree murder.

And every Sunday, the pastor of the Baptist Congregation in Erwin Tennessee, where Garland went to church as a boy, leads a prayer that "the good Lord will, according to His good will, direct Arville Garland's attorneys to do right and the good Lord, according to His will, will direct the jury to the truth."

"Most of the folks down here don't see anything wrong with

what he done," Roy Garland said. "Most of the folks down here say they would have done the same thing. I feel sorry for the parents of the boys he killed, but I don't see how hurting Arvie will help them now. He will make himself suffer enough for what he did."

———

Arville Garland was convicted of murdering the four teens. He was sentenced to ten to fifteen years for killing his daughter and ten to forty years for killing the three boys.

He spent only ten years in prison and was paroled in 1980. While in prison he received more than 1,000 letters from frustrated parents congratulating him for killing his daughter and her friends.

Garland was able to live the last twenty-four years of his life as a free man. He died in his home town of Erwin, Tennessee, when he was seventy-nine.

Chapter 3

The Catholic Church was the center of our lives where I grew up in a four-bedroom red brick house at 16903 Cheyenne St. near Six Mile Road and Schaefer in the northwest section of Detroit.

My parents were married on St. Patrick's Day in 1944. In the picture I have of their wedding, my father is dressed in an Army uniform. My mother wears a well-tailored suit. Their smiles glow off the page. Earl and Rebecca Ricke were married for sixty-eight years. My mother, who was a year older than my father, died when she was ninety-one. My father died two years later when he was ninety-two.

I am a baby boomer born in 1946 just after the war ended. I am the oldest of five children. There are nine years between me and my brother, Bernie, the youngest sibling in the family. My sisters Sue, Kathy, and Peggy came in between Bernie and me.

The Catholic compound named Precious Blood Church and Elementary School was only a block and a half from our house. The two-story school stood next to a large parking lot that served as a playground at lunchtime. Our beautiful church with stained glass windows and a colorful mosaic on the ceiling was across the street from the school.

There was a rectory where the priests lived on one side of the church. And there was a convent on the other side of the church where the Dominican nuns who taught in the school lived. School started at 8:15 each morning when the children attended mass before marching across the street to the school.

I was a sickly child with a severe case of asthma that stayed with me through my grade school years. I missed weeks of school at a time. The nuns would send work home, and my mother would go over it with me. My parents wanted me to take the third grade over because I missed so much of it, but the Dominican sisters told them I was smart enough to get by in fourth grade, and I was too young to lose a year from my life. I don't remember my grades in elementary school, but since I did very well in high school I assume the grade school report cards were pretty good.

I have many boxes that have moved with me over the years. Some have been moved from place to place without being opened for decades. Some contain layers of yellow, crisp newsprint from my career as a journalist. Then there are the speeches for the governor of New York. For years I wrote freelance speeches for Earl Graves, founder and publisher of *Black Enterprise Magazine*. There was a box filled with those speeches and a box of magazines that contained my articles. While digging through one of the older boxes, I found a Precious Blood elementary school report card. It didn't say what grade it measured, but it reported all C's and D's for me. My long absences must have affected my school work after all.

I remember struggling to catch my breath. I recall still dark nights lit by the soft yellow lights from a radio in a room filled with the smell of Vicks. I remember vomiting tons of phlegm. I remember oxygen and hospitals. The field across the street from our house was filled with weeds. I was allergic to pollen. And the allergies caused hay fever which triggered asthma. So for much of the summer vacation I was not allowed to play outside.

My father built a Lionel railroad set for me. It was on a six by five-foot table he made. It had two engines, tunnels, a station with little people inside, and a cattle car with little cows that moved from their pen to the waiting car. I spent hours and hours with those trains. Since I was not allowed outside during the hot summer, my friends would have to come to my house to play with me. The train set was a great magnet for friends.

Precious Blood Church and school were not the only Catholic influences on our lives. Two of my father's four brothers were Franciscan priests. They were stationed at a college seminary in a Detroit suburb, and I saw a lot of them. We would meet at my grandmother's house for Sunday dinner at least twice a month. They made a ceremony out of making martinis with my grandfather.

Father Peter took me fishing with my grandfather. He took me to Detroit Tiger baseball games. I listened to every game I could on my transistor radio. When I got to see them in person, I was in heaven, even if they lost.

Father Lucian taught me photography. When I was still in grade school, he helped me put together a dark room under the basement stairs.

My father bought me a nice camera. I saved up for a used enlarger. Before long I was developing my own film and enlarging my own black-and-white pictures.

At church I became an altar boy. I was a very devout and serious Catholic by the time I finished eighth grade. I said a rosary each and every day. I decided to follow my uncles' footsteps and entered the Franciscan seminary near Cincinnati, Ohio, where boys who wanted to be priests were taken for high school.

Father Lucian transferred to that seminary and ended up being our Latin teacher. There were more than sixty young men in the freshman class.

I was a good student there. I don't remember my grades, but I do remember my uncles and parents were proud of me. They let you come home for one summer and then you live with them forever. When I came home that first summer I didn't know what to do with myself. I saw an article in the paper about Red Cross volunteers in downtown Detroit. I rode the bus downtown. We had lists of people to call to ask for donations. I don't remember much about the work, but I still do remember Janet.

There were about three or four boys in this program and some fifty teenage girls. I couldn't stop thinking about Janet. I was fifteen and my voice wasn't the only thing that had changed.

I wanted to call Janet at home and ask her to go to the movies with me. I daydreamed what it would be like to kiss her. Because I was in the seminary and devoting myself to a life of absolute chastity, I was afraid these feelings were mortal sins that could send me to hell. Yet I still couldn't give them up.

Toward the end of the summer, I told my parents I had made a very difficult decision. I didn't want to go back to the seminary. I told them I thought I was too young to make a lifetime decision to give up relations with the opposite sex before I had any idea what those relationships were. I did have the wonderful example of my parents' relationship while they lovingly raised five children during their sixty-eight year marriage, but that seemed totally different to me from taking a girl to the movies and perhaps even kissing her.

My uncles, especially Father Lucian, were very disappointed. Lucian kept a picture of me on his desk for the rest of his life. I told them I could still be a priest someday when I was old enough to make that serious of a decision.

I took Janet to the movies. I was too young to drive, so my father drove us there and picked us up after the movie was over.

I enrolled in the Jesuit University of Detroit High School. They put me in classical studies where you studied Latin and Greek along with typical high school subjects.

I loved every minute of high school. For the most part, the asthma kept quiet.

Perhaps because I came from the seminary, it seemed to me that the Jesuits took a special interest in my life. They suggested I become a trainer for the school's football and basketball teams. I took a special course in the summer, and I ended up traveling with the teams for every game. I would tape their ankles and help prepare them for the games. I sat on the bench with them. I got to wear the teams' letters on my school sweater.

Because of my years sick with asthma when I was a virtual prisoner in my house, I felt very different from other kids. In high school all of that changed. We had sock hops every Friday night. I was popular. I had lots of friends. I had no problem finding dates. I was in the honors program and I graduated second in my class with a 95 percent average. I studied very hard at home each evening. I bet I averaged two hours each night on homework and studying for the next day's class. And I probably averaged at least half an hour on the phone each evening. After all, this was forty years before cell phones.

One day toward the end of my senior year I was called to the principal's office where I met a priest from Xavier College in Cincinnati, Ohio. They told me I could have a full scholarship that would cover everything including room, board, and tuition. I would live in a special mansion that housed students in the honors program. It required twenty-one hours of accelerated courses each semester. You had to take courses amounting to a double major, one in classical studies (Latin and Greek) and another of your choice. All the classes were accelerated honors classes and you had to earn at least a 3.3 grade point average to keep the scholarship. Talk it over with your parents, they said, and let them know whether I wanted to take advantage of the wonderful offer.

I gladly accepted the scholarship. It would be my second year away from home, both times in Cincinnati. My father and mother left my sisters and brother with my grandparents and drove a station wagon filled with me and my stuff to Xavier University.

We drove to the honor-student housing in the old mansion. In my room there were four of us in two bunk beds. Each of us had a desk, a dresser, and a small closet for our clothes.

My first strong memory of college that year was not an academic one. It was a party called "drink or drown." The young men and women paid a couple of bucks allowing them to drink as much beer as they could keep down.

In those days in Ohio, you could drink what was called 3.2 beer if you were 18. That weak beer gave me my first high, my first wonderful feelings from alcohol. I loved it. Nothing in my life up to then, except religion, made me feel so good. I wouldn't know for another thirty years that I was self-medicating for an illness I didn't know I had.

From that night on, I told myself I would study hard during the week and party hard on weekend evenings. The beer didn't change my life all that much. I still studied. I still went to class. I still wanted to excel. And I still wanted to drink, really wanted to drink. When I was in high school, I studied and felt confident of my ongoing academic success. I had a great teenage social life. I still believed strongly in the Catholic Church.

In college something changed. There were times when I could stay up all night studying and ace my tests. And there were times I felt sad and lonely even though I lived in a house full of young men.

At the time, I had no idea what was happening to me. I knew I felt out of sorts. I blamed the feelings on being away from home. I blamed the anxiety on the heavy academic load I was carrying. Even in high school when I was doing so well, I felt different than I thought others felt. But times were good then, very good, and who was I to argue with social and academic success? I was a million miles away from Precious Blood and unable to play outside with the other kids.

In the honors program at Xavier University I felt like I was drowning. I felt like I was a failure except when I was drinking. Then I felt on top of the world.

My roommates seemed to get the academics easier and better than me. But they also studied longer and harder than I did. And I continued to drink more than they did. There was a grownup bar at the end of our block. I looked older than I was and they served me adult drinks there.

So I used to walk down to the bar once in a while, desperate for the magic potion that would either slow me down or make me feel better, or both.

At the time I thought I was taking the easy way out from under a huge load of difficult schoolwork. Keeping up with twenty-one hours of tough honors courses was no easy task no matter how long or hard you studied.

I wasn't a raving drunk. Drinking during the week was an exception. I did study most weekday nights. But I loved that 3.2 beer on weekends. I had a girlfriend from the neighboring Catholic girls' college. I should have been happier. I should have felt I was having a good life. My college was paid for. I had friends at school. I had a girlfriend. But, as time went by, I had a growing fear that I wasn't smart enough for the honors program. I was miserable at times. And I didn't seem to care enough about grades and studying even when I felt on top of the world.

At the end of the school year, the priest whose job it was to take care of the honors students called me down to his office on the first floor of the mansion. My fears were realized when he told me my grades were not good enough to continue in the honors program. My grade-point average was around 2.8. They could have made an exception, he told me, but my extra-curricular social life tipped the scale against me. I could come back to Xavier and take regular classes but I would have to pay for them myself. I was stunned. It was the first academic failure of my life, and it authenticated all my feelings of being different from others, of not being good enough.

My parents were rich with love and attention for their five children. But raising five children cost every cent my father took home. My father got me a summer job on the assembly line making Mustangs. I was a spot welder.

The cars would come speeding by, one a minute or so, and I would have to use my big, bulky, heavy welding gun to put a bunch of welds on the cars. Keeping up was very difficult for me. At times, I missed some welds. But no one said anything. That line of half-built cars kept on coming and coming no matter what. The emphasis in those days was quantity over quality. Never stop that line. At night when I lay in my bed, I could feel it moving just like the line. Today welding machines do all of that work.

I made enough during the summers to pay much of my tuition. During the school year, I worked some evenings delivering booze and beer for the corner liquor store. I enrolled at the University of Detroit (U of D), a Jesuit university about three miles from my house. I only had to take fifteen hours or fewer of regular courses. School was a breeze here compared to Xavier's honors program.

My interest in photography led me to the *Varsity News*, U of D's official newspaper. I volunteered to be a photographer. As I was taking and developing pictures for the *Varsity News*, I got to know the reporters and editors of the paper. The students who majored in journalism were a tight-knit group. They attended classes together. They put out the school newspaper, and they traveled to high schools to hold journalism classes focused on the writing and production of high school papers. I signed up for the program. I put my camera down and became a reporter. After a year or so, I got a job putting out a weekly bulletin for a nearby Catholic church, St. Cecelia. I wrote the articles, took the pictures and put it all together.

For my social life outside of the journalism department, I became a member of TKE, a fraternity with a house on campus where the weekend parties were legendary.

Most of us weren't twenty-one yet, but we still drank a lot. Weekends at the TKE house were Detroit's version of Cincinnati's drink-and-drowns. I continued to live at home until I graduated from college. Eventually I became editor of the *Varsity News*.

Neil Shine, a great newspaperman who was the city editor of the *Detroit Free Press* at the time, was a graduate of U of D's journalism program. One thing led to another and the *Free Press* hired me as a copyboy when I was a junior in college. This was before word processors and personal computers. Every story for the paper was typed on antique Underwood typewriters. The reporters typed on six layers of thin paper separated by sheets of carbon paper that were called "books." In order to make impressions on each of the six pages, you had to really pound the keys.

Different editors got copies of the stories. There was a city desk for local stories, and another desk for national stories that used material from Knight Ridder's Washington, DC, office, national correspondents, and both the Associated Press (AP) and United Press International (UPI).

The news editor laid out the paper, deciding where each article would be placed. Some had to be cut to fit into their prearranged space.

The final stop was the copy desk, a large circular desk where editors read the stories one last time and wrote headlines to fit on top of them.

Copyboys ran around delivering all the copies of the stories from desk to desk in the news room. We tore off stories from the clacking AP and UPI wire machines and delivered them to the right editors. We did a lot of errands.

We were forever going downstairs where there was a restaurant on the first floor of the *Free Press* building to get coffee for the news staff. Yells of "Copy, copy, copy!" became more frequent and fierce as the final deadlines approached.

Copyboys wrote the short weather briefs every day, and that was the most coveted assignment. There's nothing quite like seeing your words in newsprint even if it was just a few words about the weather.

Chapter 4

I don't recall exactly how long I was a copyboy. I do remember the summer college interns, young men and women our age who worked as junior reporters while we fetched them coffee. There was a pecking order in the newsroom. Copyboys were definitely on the bottom rung of the editorial employee ladder. I was one of the copyboys who was a college student majoring in journalism just like the summer interns.

Even though it seemed unfair to the college student copyboys to make them wait on the college student interns, copyboys who wanted to be reporters really had the upper hand. The newspaper guild union contract stipulated that under certain circumstances copyboys had to be given a six-month tryout to become a reporter. There were limited openings for new reporters. As a very interested copyboy, I had real hope for a future in journalism. The *Detroit Free Press* had a popular front-page feature called "Action Line." It was a column that answered readers' questions and used the power of the press to solve issues for them with companies and government agencies. I was promoted from copyboy to researcher for Action Line. Just after I graduated from college I was promoted again. Now I was a reporter. Looking back at all my work over the years, that was probably the job I enjoyed the most.

I started on the police beat. You had to read reams of police reports looking for the ones that would be newsworthy, looking for the ones with white people involved.

If black people were involved in crimes, newspapers in those days wouldn't cover much of it unless it was really sensational.

On the police beat you didn't write stories yourself very often. You phoned the facts into a rewrite man and he wrote the story based on your reporting.

After the police beat, I covered the courts. Two of my biggest ongoing stories were court cases—Arville Garland and James Johnson, Jr. I did in-depth feature stories on the big story cases before the trials and then covered the trials writing stories based on the testimony of the day. If it was a big deal trial, my stories often made the front page.

While I was busy gaining professional stature as a staff writer, I was also gaining a lot of weight. I still was a big drinker. After work I would go the Detroit Press Club for drinks and sometimes dinner. I favored bourbon manhattans at the press club and beer from the tap at Leo's Anchor Bar where I often went after the Press Club closed.

I weighed about 210 when I joined the *Free Press*. I was six-two so I looked like a stocky football player. Over the months and years, I kept gaining weight until I weighed over 300 pounds. I wrote many of my best stories when I was obese. I had good friends in the business. I didn't think anyone could like me because of my appearance. People who were my friends had to be motivated by my work. They must have liked me because they liked the stories I wrote.

Tom Wark was my favorite editor. Whenever he would edit a story of mine it would come out better, but he was more than an editor to me.

He became my mentor and my good friend. We would hang out and talk shop at Press Club.

I was surprised one day when he called me over to his desk in the city room and asked me to sit down. He told me that everyone was noticing my heavy drinking and my outlandish life style. I needed help, he said, especially help with my drinking. He gave me a slip of paper with the name and phone number of a psychologist who specialized in alcoholism. Either see this man, he told me, or you will lose your job.

I started to see him and that relationship started my lifetime involvement with mental health professionals.

In the last half of my six years with the *Free Press*, I wrote many lead articles for the front page of the Sunday feature section. I wrote a lot of stories for the *Sunday Magazine*. I wrote front page news stories. I was becoming a very good journalist—a resourceful and sensitive reporter and an excellent writer. I don't want to sound like I'm bragging, but I was really good at my job back then. I lived a double life, good at my work during the day and lost in an alcohol-fueled search for human companionship at night.

I met Judy one night at the Detroit Press Club. She was having dinner by herself. I don't remember how I managed it, but I ended up having dinner with her. Judy was a very pretty blonde who was really smart and somewhat unsure of herself. We became friends over the next few months, good friends. She was engaged to a nice thin guy who liked to drink.

There were days when I didn't drink. But when I drank, I drank. The psychologist I was seeing told me I could be an episodic alcoholic. I guess that meant I was only an alcoholic when I drank, when I would stay at the bar until it closed at two a.m.

I didn't drink so much all of the time, but sometimes when I did, it would slow my racing brain down and make me feel stupid.

Alcohol was most dangerous when I was depressed. It added fuel to the pain and despair. It would take two decades before I would be told my substance abuse was another symptom of my bipolar disorder because I was really self-medicating for the sharp ups and dismal downs of the illness.

Judy and I started to have good times together. We went to the movies. We went out to dinner. We went drinking. I took her to Tange's to show her the underbelly of the city. We saw each other frequently right from the start. Sometimes when her fiancé wasn't around, I would hang out at the Anchor bar until she finished her shift so that we could have a few drinks together. During this time, I was unwittingly building my reputation as a real character with journalistic talent. At some point, we crossed the line and slept together. Because I was so heavy, I feared she would think she made a mistake and turn what happened into a one-night stand. Instead our relationship became romantic. We saw each other all of the time. I couldn't believe my good fortune. She ditched her fiancé and married me instead. To me it was like beauty and the beast.

During the first couple years of our marriage, my life improved dramatically. Every newspaper reporters' dream is to have a book published.

An editor from Bantam Books gave me a contract to write a book on the outcome of a trial I covered for the paper. I was paid a year's salary as an advance to write a book about the case of James Johnson, Jr. Johnson was part of the largest migration in US history. He abandoned plantation life in Starkville, Mississippi, to travel to Detroit, Michigan, where a man could make a very good living working in the auto plants.

Equal opportunity was not doing so well in the auto industry. Johnson worked at menial, low-paying jobs not in the auto industry for more than fifteen years. Then his dream finally came true and he got a good-paying job at a Chrysler plant in Detroit.

One summer day halfway through a shift, his foreman fired him. Johnson returned to the plant with a gun. He shot and killed three white foremen. It looked like an open-and-shut case of triple homicide. There were scores of witnesses who saw Johnson kill his bosses.

Two young attorneys defended Johnson. Kenneth Cockrel and Justin Ravitz made the case into an indictment of the entire auto industry. They convinced the nearly all-white jury that the racist way Johnson was treated in the auto plant made him legally insane and not criminally responsible for the killings.

I called the book *Blood on a Northern Plantation*. It took me a year to report and write it. This was the early seventies and power to the people, indiscriminate sex, long hair, marijuana, and bell bottom pants were becoming middle class.

I didn't get along all that well with the *Free Press*'s executive editor, Kurt Luedke. Only the publisher had more clout.

We talked from time to time. But I wasn't one of his people. I was one of Tom Wark's people. Because I felt he didn't like me I underestimated his talent. I told myself Luedke was an empty suit who knew little about writing. I was so wrong about his talent. Luedke left the paper to write movies. The first one he wrote was *Absence of Malice.* Then he wrote *Out of Africa.* He won an Academy Award. That took a lot more talent than I thought I would ever have.

I took a leave of absence from the *Free Press* to write the book on James Johnson. Bantam divided the process into thirds. Each time I finished a third of the book, I would receive a third of the advance.

I joined Weight Watchers, and with Judy's support and encouragement I stuck with it for more than a year. I followed the diet like a religion. I quit drinking except for a very occasional glass of white wine. I lost more than 100 pounds and kept it off. I was on the cover of *Weight Watchers Magazine* and the *Detroit Free Press Sunday Magazine* wearing the old pants, holding the empty waist out in front of me.

I got a call from Laird Harris, who was the campaign manager for Sandy Levin who was running for governor of Michigan. Harris offered me the job of director of communications for the campaign. I took the temporary assignment instead of going back to the *Free Press.* Sandy Levin was a terrific guy. The congressman was serious and smart and he really knew how to get along with people. He is the brother of Carl Levin who has been a US senator from Michigan forever.

The most crucial part of a political campaign is raising money and putting blockbuster commercials on TV. David Garth, along with his associates, Jeff Greenfield and Maureen Connolly, produced Levin's television commercials and set the public tone of the campaign. I wrote press releases. I also worked with Greenfield on speeches.

He had been a speechwriter for Bobby Kennedy when he was practically a child. He was one of the best in the business.

Garth was doing two campaigns that season, Sandy Levin for governor of Michigan and Hugh Carey for governor of New York.

I was paid for my work on the campaign. Judy helped out when she could as a volunteer. Once the campaign started moving, I was rarely home at a decent hour. There were always press releases to write, reporters from print, radio, and TV to talk to, issues to understand and speeches to write. Greenfield wrote the campaign stump speeches that could be used over and over. I would tailor Greenfield's speeches to specific audiences. And I eventually got to the point where I would write speeches myself. I loved writing speeches, writing to be heard not read. Writing with a rhythm, writing with feeling and facts mixed together like oratorical music.

Despite a well-run campaign, a talented and dedicated staff, enough money to put excellent commercials on television, despite everything good Levin stood for, we lost the election. Our opponent, incumbent governor William Milliken, was extremely popular. And, despite how critical we were about him during the campaign, looking back he certainly wasn't a bad governor.

Garth's other candidate, Congressman Hugh Carey, won his election to be governor of New York.

After the concession statement was history and the offices were cleared out, I got a call from Greenfield. Would I be interested in writing speeches for Hugh Carey?

Being chief speechwriter for the governor of New York was fuel for my ego. It was a better job than I would have been offered if Levin had won, simply because it was in New York. I flew to New York City for an interview. I met with Greenfield, Garth, and Connolly. And I interviewed with David Burke, Carey's brilliant chief of staff who also had worked for the Kennedys.

Because Garth and Greenfield vouched for me, I had the inside track for the job. I couldn't believe my good fortune; I was offered a six-month tryout to be chief speechwriter for the governor of New York, which is probably the writing capital of the world. I would spend half of my time in the state capital, Albany, and the other half in midtown Manhattan where the governor had an office. I would have to go wherever the governor went.

The six-month tryout would also be a trial for our marriage. Because I was on a tryout with no guarantee that I would have a permanent position, Judy and I decided that she should stay in Detroit and keep her job until we knew what the outcome of my tryout would be. We would get together whenever we could, but neither of us realized how infrequent that would be.

Before he was elected governor, Carey had been a congressman from Brooklyn for many years. As governor, Carey was leading the public charge to save New York City from defaulting on its securities. Just about every time he gave an address, he made the case for the federal government to guarantee his city's securities. Saving New York City wouldn't cost the government a dime. And a New York City default would have disastrous national consequences. All Washington had to do was guarantee the city's securities, and New York would make massive cuts and be able to afford to pay what it owed investors.

Those who were against the federal government helping the city said New York spent way beyond its means for many years. Now it was time for the city to get what it deserved, bankruptcy.

President Gerald Ford decided not to guarantee New York City's securities thinking that national public opinion would be against the city. The famous *New York Daily News* headline, "Ford to City: Drop Dead" began to demonstrate how Ford's decision would backfire.

When I joined his staff, Governor Carey was in the middle of the save the city campaign. I began to write his speeches.

The first few weren't bad, but he didn't want to say something the same way twice in his speeches. If a line worked for one speech, he would rather not use it again in the next speech. At least that's the way I remember it.

After all this happened forty-five years ago. This was way

before personal computers. I typed the speech on a special IBM electric typewriter with large type. I would mark corrections and edits made by others in pencil and my secretary would produce the final product.

I recently reread many of the speeches I kept copies of during my two years on the job, from 1974 to 1976. They are better than I remembered. Most of them concerned the precarious financial situation for New York City and state and the urgent need for deep cuts in city and state spending. For many years, New York City and state, where one-tenth of America's citizens lived, led the nation in spending for new government programs. New York now had to lead in the cutting and scaling back of programs. And it was my job to convince everyone why "the days of wine and roses" were over in New York, and to convince them how necessary this new fiscal restraint was for the city and state's future.

Even though I was surrounded by loyal and talented Carey staffers, I felt alone in the demanding professional situation. Carey was a very difficult customer for any speechwriter. He was 100 percent Irish through and through and loved the sound and power of words. He did not like the first drafts of a number of my speeches.

I began to drink on weekends in Manhattan. Then I drank in Albany where I eventually got an apartment. For the first two months or so, I lived in hotels. The state had vouchers I used to pay for the rooms.

During much of my success at the Detroit Free Press I weighed 300 pounds and women looked the other way. Now, at twenty-seven, I was the governor of New York's chief speechwriter. And I weighed a trim 185. Despite my recent good looks, despite my influential job at the tender age of twenty-seven, inside I still felt somewhat fat and inferior. I often felt I was in over my head. However, I soon noticed that women looked at me differently than they did when I was fat. And it was the first time in my adult life that women flirted with me and strongly hinted that we should be together, at least for that night.

Women had never looked at me that way before. When I gave

in, it was good for my exploding ego, but, of course, bad for my marriage. As far as I know Judy never found out about it.

My life became a blur of traveling back and forth between New York City and Albany. The more pressure-packed the job became, the more I drank. At first I didn't drink while I was writing a speech, a process that could last for days. Before long, I would drink a couple on the nights between days of writing. There was a bar in Albany within walking distance of the capital called The Assembly where I used to hang out with some elected officials and their staffs. I was somebody there, I was the governor's speech-writer, and I was very young for a job like that.

I flew home on a few weekends when I was in between speeches and could take a break. When my mother was ninety years old she had a terrific memory.

She reminded me of a time when Judy went to the airport and discovered I wasn't on the plane I was supposed to be on. Apparently, according to my mother, I missed a second flight and ended up not coming home at all that weekend. Judy then told my mom that I wasn't the same person after I lost weight. And she was right.

I think Judy was getting used to not having me around and liked living by herself. From time to time she would tell me she didn't like being married anymore. I couldn't stand the thought of losing her so I didn't take her seriously when she complained about being married. There were two huge speeches I had to write for the governor each year.

One was the State of New York address to the legislature that was heavily covered by the press. And there is a ton of media in New York, including the *New York Times, Newsday, The New York Post,* and the *Daily News,* not to mention all the radio and television stations. New York's precarious fiscal situation had become national news during the tough economic times of the middle seventies.

The second big speech of the year was the governor's annual State of the Health speech that Carey originated. Carey's wife, Helen, had died before he became governor, leaving him with a house filled with children to raise on his own. The doctor who cared for Helen Carey was Dr. Kevin Cahill. No one was closer to the governor than Dr. Cahill. His title was Special Assistant to the Governor for Health Affairs. It was Dr. Cahill who persuaded his friend to give the health address.

David Burke made my speeches better, and I learned from his suggestions. Carey gave my speeches somewhat close to the way I had written them, including the very long address to the legislature. But preparing those speeches was still a grueling process.

I did have what I thought would be terrific news. I finally got in touch with the editor from Bantam Books who handled my James Johnson Book, *Blood on a Northern Plantation*.

We went to lunch in a midtown Manhattan restaurant. The bottom line was they were not going to publish it. I could keep the advance and I would have the rights to the book back, but the project wasn't going anywhere at Bantam. I asked him if something was wrong with my reporting or writing or the point of view I took in writing the book.

After all, I reminded him, Bantam had sent me checks after I sent in each third of the book. Why all of a sudden was it an inferior product now? It was partially a marketing decision, he said, these types of books aren't selling very well now.

I felt devastated. Having the book published was my most urgent professional dream. It was more important to me than any other professional endeavor, including writing speeches for Governor Carey. But I didn't have too much time to lick my wounds; there was always another speech to write.

After my tryout was over Judy would take her time joining me as she debated whether or not she wanted to be married anymore. It got to the point where when someone would ask me if I was married, I would think I would have to call Judy to find out.

My drinking continued.

I had my favorite places in the city. P.J. Clarke's was one of them. I discovered after-hours clubs both in New York City and Albany.

Occasionally I broke my rule about not drinking while I was writing. Sometimes when I wrote the speeches I was quick and focused and firmly in control of my work. At those times I felt like I was writing music. Then there were other times when I worked slow as molasses, forcing one word to come after another.

Judy finally quit her job in Michigan and joined me in New York. After some time in Albany she wanted a separation. I was doubly devastated. First my book. Now my marriage. She wanted to live on her own in the city. While Judy was enjoying her new job in Manhattan, I was still traveling back and forth between the state capital and the big city writing speeches for the governor.

One night when a convention was in town, the hotels that took state vouchers were fully booked and I couldn't find a room. I called Judy and asked if she would put me up for a night in the apartment I was still paying for. I offered to sleep on the couch. She refused me, and I was so angry and drunk I smashed the phone booth glass with the receiver and drove my state car back to Albany, struggling to drive while intoxicated. The more I couldn't see her, the more I wanted to be with her. I fluctuated between being very alert and angry to being very depressed and lonely. Judy had finally agreed to meet me after she got off work at nine that evening. We were to meet in her apartment.

I tried to be optimistic. Maybe this meeting would be good. I was flooded with anxiety. Would we get back together? Would this be the permanent end of the marriage? I would know in a couple of hours.

Soon I was pulling up in a cab in front of her apartment building. There was a bottle of Jack Daniels, my favorite drink in those days, on the kitchen table. I had a baggie of grass in my pocket. I was looking forward to getting high with Judy and solving our problems.

Hours passed and there was still no sign of Judy. I decided I might as well have a drink or two while I waited. Sometimes she had to work late. I called her office, and no one answered.

The pain was growing deeper and deeper. Where could she be? It was now past midnight, and still no sign of her. I continued to drink. Then I smoked dope and kept drinking. I was getting really stoned, and the higher I got the more it hurt.

I heard her in the hallway.

"Where have you been?" I said. "I have been waiting for you all night."

"None of your fucking business," she replied, and I took a swing at her.

She dropped her bag of groceries and ran to her neighbors' apartment.

I knew my marriage was over for good, and I was more depressed than ever before. I was being dragged across a field of barbed wire and broken glass. I had never hurt this bad before. I was dying with overpowering grief from the breakup of our marriage.

I was bleeding inside my soul. How could I stop this? I would do anything to stop the pain. Anything. I put my hand in my pocket and pulled out a full bottle of Elavil. (I must have been seeing a doctor who prescribed the psychotropic medicine for me. I don't remember.) I knew what I was going to do. I couldn't bear the thought of living on my own without Judy. Although she never found out, I was overpowered by guilt for being unfaithful to her. Judy was gone, and I didn't want to live without her. I couldn't stand this pain. I would do anything to end it. It seemed like I was a total failure in life. My book would never be published. I could never really please the governor, and I could never really please my wife. Neither of them really wanted me.

I was looking at the bottle of Elavil in my hand, and I knew now what I was going to do.

I started taking the pills, one by one, washing them down with the whiskey. I longed for the sweet nothingness of death. I longed for this pain to end. There would be nothing at all after that, and it would be like before I was born. Nothing.

Or there would be an afterlife, and God would understand my pain and allow me into heaven. Either way would be better than all of this pain I had. I kept taking the pills until they were all gone. Then I had to write a note, a farewell note for Judy.

I wrote that my passing was all her fault. I told her I couldn't stand the pain she put me in. And I told her that now she could be happy without me.

I kept waiting for something to happen, and I was still okay. I was drunk and high, but nothing was happening from the Elavil. I read my suicide note again and tore it up. I wrote another note, and I told her that I wanted to die to end the pain in my life, but it wasn't her fault.

People break up every day, and they don't commit suicide. *I am different*, I wrote, *and I must do this. You know you are better off without me.*

I heard a knocking on the door. It was our neighbor, Tim. He came over to see how I was doing. He saw the empty bottle of pills on the coffee table. He saw the suicide note. He read it.

"Tom, let's go to the hospital," he said.

"No way," I replied. "Nothing is going to happen, Tim. It's been over an hour since I took those pills, and nothing is happening to me. I don't need to go to the hospital."

"You have a choice," Tim answered, "either you come to the hospital with me, or I will call the police. I'm serious. It's your choice."

We were on the way to the hospital in Tim's car when we stopped at a red light.

There was a bar glowing with neon to our left.

"Tim, I don't need to go to the hospital," I said. "Nothing is happening. Let's stop and have a beer and talk about this. That will help me more than the hospital."

Tim looked at the bar. He looked at the empty pill bottle he put on the dashboard. "No," he said, "any other time I would stop, but not now."

We pulled up at the emergency room entrance to the hospital. Tim and I walked into the emergency room. After a few steps, I fell flat on my face. Two nurses ran out to where I was lying on the floor. I was unconscious and having difficulty breathing.

Chapter 5

When I awoke a few days later, I could not remember what had happened. I was obviously in a hospital. And as I began to sit up a little and look around, I saw my parents sitting near the end of my bed.

At first, I didn't know why I was in a hospital and why my parents were there. A couple of nurses and a doctor came running in after my parents told them I was awake. I didn't know why everyone seemed so happy.

"Mr. Ricke," the doctor said, "you have just come out of a deep coma. We thought we may have lost you."

I don't remember much about my stay in the hospital that saved my life. I remember being in a large room with several young people who were there for abnormal behavior from abuse of drugs. I still have the image of a group of teenage girls huddled in a corner listening to Barry White's "Can't Get Enough of Your Love, Babe" over and over while their hips gently rocked back and forth to the rhythm of the music.

What I remember most about my stay in that hospital was Judy's visit. She came to see me with papers in her hand. "I know this isn't all your fault," she said. "Both of us put you here." She said she was sorry for the way she had treated me. She said she wanted us to be together. She put some papers in front of me. "You need help," she said. "You need to go to another hospital."

She asked me to sign papers that would commit me to a psychiatric ward in a Manhattan hospital where I would probably stay for at least a month.

She told me what happened had been her fault too. She told me she would visit me in the hospital and take part in my therapy. When I got out, she said, we would live together and get further help. I couldn't believe what I was hearing. We would be back together again, and it would be like the early days of our marriage when we were so happy together.

I didn't hesitate. I signed the papers.

She didn't come to visit. In fact, I would only see her again when we met to discuss terms of the divorce months after I was released from the hospital.

My parents had to go home after a while. The only visitor I remember having in the psychiatric unit was Jeff Greenfield. I was touched by his visit. He wanted to see how I was doing. He knew how difficult it could be to write for the New York governor. He wanted to know if working for Carey had driven me to my suicide attempt. He said he felt responsible for bringing me to the Carey administration. I agreed that Governor Carey could be difficult to work for, but I told Greenfield I really admired how Carey had a huge role in saving New York City from default and bankruptcy. I had very painful marital problems, I told Greenfield, and those painful issues were the catalyst for the psychotic episode that nearly killed me, not Carey. I also told him I thought there was something else going on with me.

People endured broken marriages all of the time, but they don't try to kill themselves. The hospital told me I might be an alcoholic. I accepted that. I certainly could drink heavily when I drank. But I wondered if there was something else going on with me.

I knew I could get very depressed even when I was sober. And there were nights I couldn't sleep, even when I wasn't on an all-night drinking spree.

Later in his life, Greenfield had an on-air television career. Every time I would see him as a commentator, I would feel grateful for his visit when I was really down and out.

Judy filed for divorce. I didn't fight it. I believed she was the cause of all the trouble in my life. I still loved her and hated her at the same time.

I would have to fall in love with someone else before I could get over her. Despite the way she ended it, when I think of Judy today, I think of her fondly. I hope she is happy wherever she is and whomever she is with.

For a few weeks after I left the hospital, I lived in a cheap, run-down hotel in Manhattan where mentally ill people were sent. I wasn't broke. A distant relative had left me and my brother and sisters several thousand dollars each. Tim found me a great apartment on the Upper West Side. His wife was an interior decorator. With her help, I had an apartment I was proud to show to guests.

The closest grocery store was around the corner on Broadway. I used a pull cart to bring groceries home. I lived on the third floor of a building with a doorman and elevator. A medium-sized black-haired dog followed me home from the grocery one day.

I noticed him because he was walking on three legs. One of his back legs was folded under him and it would only come down occasionally. The third time he followed me home, I let him follow me inside and decided to keep him. I named him Sunshine and he stayed with me for another nine years.

As I fully expected, I lost my job at the governor's office. They came and got the state car. There was no "You're fired, get out of here." I knew they didn't want me back after what happened. So I didn't try to go back.

I was trying to sell my book when I met Gay Hege, a literary agent who had been a book editor at Doubleday and was just starting a business on her own. She loved my book and said she was confident she could get it published.

She would go out to dinner quite often with a small group of writers and friends.

I became one of the group. I was grateful to have this social life and the friends who came along with it. I mostly didn't drink. But I smoked grass when I could get it.

Even when I wasn't drinking I would occasionally stay up all night and go to after-hours clubs and drink Cokes. After about six months of not working, I got a call from Mike O'Neill, the editor of the *New York Daily News*. He wanted me to come to his office and meet with him. I didn't know why he wanted to see me. He was a terrific guy who was on a mission to improve the editorial quality of the tabloid with screaming headlines.

He said he had talked to Carey's office and had called Detroit to ask about me, and he wanted to find out if I was interested in being a "newspaperman" again. He asked me what I would like to do at his newspaper. I was silent for a while.

I didn't answer him right away. He told me it seemed to him I didn't have any specific career goals, that I didn't know what I wanted to do with my life. I told him there were a lot of things I could do at the *Daily News*, but I didn't want to be considered a candidate for one specific job. What if I said I wanted to be a sportswriter and you already had those positions filled? What if I said I wanted to be a columnist but you didn't need anyone else now that you had Jimmy Breslin and Pete Hamill?

I asked him where he needed help. I told him I would like to work somewhere in the paper where I could make a difference. He told me he was looking for help on the editorial page. He was looking for someone with a keen understanding of city and state government, someone who was an expert on the new era of cutbacks in New York government. When he brought up my hospitalization, I said, "You would hire a person with a broken arm if it was healing. My situation isn't much different."

I told him I would love to write editorials for the *Daily News*, a paper with a circulation in the millions at the time. I suggested a tryout. He would have nothing to lose that way. If I didn't cut the mustard in a reasonable amount of time, I would just leave.

We agreed on a tryout. I would start right away working with editor Jack Smee and writers Don McCormick and Henry Lee on the editorial board of the paper.

Writing editorials for the *Daily News* was the most difficult writing challenge I had ever experienced. I was used to writing long feature stories for magazines or speeches that would last twenty minutes or more. The majority of the editorials were very short. You had three or four paragraphs to define an issue, take a position on it, and close gracefully. On more complex issues you might have five or six paragraphs to work with.

Once in a while, a whole column would be devoted to a single subject. But not often. We had editorial board meetings every morning. O'Neill presided over the meetings and Smee would guide us through the rest of the day before O'Neill saw the final versions.

Those short, punchy editorials packed a lot of power. The governor, Mayor Ed Koch, and the state's US Senators and Representatives would visit us to ask support for one program or another. We also saw prominent people from Washington, the United Nations, and the private sector. They all wanted the *Daily News* editorial board to see things their way.

We tended to specialize in certain areas. Because I knew something about city and state government and had my sources for information—people I used to work with—I started writing editorials about city and state government issues. I remember the first time Carey visited us. He stared at me as if to say, "What is he doing here?"

I found out later that Dr. Cahill was interested in what happened to me. He understood that mental health problems were not a person's fault any more than cancer or heart disease. Once you found out you had the behavioral illness, it was your responsibility to get care, take the prescribed medicines, and follow medical instructions, but getting it in the first place was a matter of genetics and fate.

Mario Cuomo, who was Secretary of State and would be governor someday, also took an interest in me. And someone told me Jimmy Breslin had his hand in what was happening on my behalf. Somehow they persuaded O'Neill to take a look at me.

Part of my responsibility was to write editorials on health care and New York City hospital issues. I also wrote editorials that were close to O'Neill and Breslin and Carey and Cahill's hearts—editorials on the situation in Northern Ireland.

I passed my tryout. Writing for a newspaper came second nature to me.

There was a lot happening at the city desk during my first summer on the new job. The Son of Sam was killing young couples in parked cars, scaring the hell out of the entire city. He wrote notes to Breslin. It was very much a *Daily News* story. I got to talk with Caroline Kennedy that summer. She was a copy girl at the *News*.

At times I felt I was on top of the world. I had a job where I earned respect. It could be difficult at times, but it was easier to please O'Neill than Hugh Carey. Carey was a very decent man, a good father, and a good governor. It was just difficult to write for him.

Another Carey alumnus joined our editorial board. Bob Laird had been Carey's press secretary when I was the chief speechwriter. At first his arrival made me insecure. I thought I was the in-house expert on state government. Had I failed? Was I not good enough? Did O'Neill have to bring in someone else with an intimate experience with local government because I didn't meet his expectations? But there was plenty of work for both of us. We became good friends and continued our friendship for many years.

So I had a really good job where what I wrote could persuade public officials on what course to take in difficult situations. My writing editorials could make a difference in public policy. My job also could be a magnet for meeting interesting women.

Despite the mass transit that could get you everywhere in New York City, I had a Mustang left over from my previous life in Detroit. I kept it in a garage in Harlem. It would stay there for months without me driving it. I would use it to get away on the weekends. A friend had a summer house with an indoor swimming pool in the Hamptons and he would let me use it from time to time.

Despite all that was good in my life, I would still get extremely depressed at times. It was harder to write then, but I could force the words to come. They came slowly and uncomfortably. My work was not as good when I was like this. During some of these sad times, I thought about suicide, thought about it a lot. On the surface my life was very good, as good as ever, but I still could be very troubled and depressed.

John Hume came to visit the *Daily News* one day. He led a popular Catholic movement in Northern Ireland called the SDLP that had nothing to do with the IRA. Ireland's government was supporting Hume's movement in the North. It was paying his way for a trip to the United Nations where he was going to speak. Ted Smyth was the official from Ireland I used to talk to about the problems in the North. In essence he was a public relations person for the government of Ireland.

We had lunch occasionally and enjoyed each other's company. He invited me to a cocktail party for Hume, a party to let UN people get to know there were Catholics for peace in Northern Ireland. The violent IRA had plenty of financial support from lads from New York City who could never get over the old violent atrocities of the British over there. Hume wanted the Catholics in the North to have a strong legal voice in the government, but he wanted to support power-sharing by non-violent means.

I took a date to the cocktail party, a woman I had recently met at another cocktail party. We got into the elevator with a tall, striking blonde whose eyes locked onto my eyes. Her name was Maura and she worked for the Irish Mission to the United Nations.

I practically ignored my date and spent as much time as I could talking with Maura. The next day I invited her to lunch. We went to a Chinese restaurant called Peng's. When it was time for the fortune cookies, I took her fortune and wrote on the back of it, "You are about to become involved with a tall writer with a mustache." She carried that piece of paper in her wallet for more than twenty years.

I did hurt Maura once in the beginning. I took another

woman I had dated before I met Maura to the summer house for a weekend. Maura cried. I stopped seeing anyone else.

Whenever we had spare time, we tried to enjoy it together. When we would spend the night together, it would be at my place because she had two Irish roommates at her apartment. I bought her a bicycle for her birthday, and we rode in Central Park and took long walks together.

We saw movies and went to the theatre and frequented popular restaurants. Sometimes when we weren't together I would drink too much and call her early in the morning. Instead of seeing these calls as a warning signal, she thought they were romantic.

We began to fall in love with each other right away. Now when I was energized and became the life of the party, I had someone who would appreciate the mood I was in. I had a great woman, apartment and job. But even when my life was going so well, I still got depressed from time to time. When I was like this, Maura told me she wanted to wrap me in the "cotton wool" of her affection.

Maura was Irish, not Irish American. She left Ireland to work for an Irish official in the UN. I loved her Irish accent and what I used to call the Irish twinkle in her eyes.

We married six months after we met in the United Nations chapel by a judge I knew from my work at the *Daily News*. Maura wanted the chapel because the picture she would send home would look like we were married in a church. And her family would assume it was a Catholic church.

We had a reception dinner at the Top of the Sixes where we could see the sparkling lights of the city below us. My family came to the wedding and reception.

We lived in my apartment. I continued my therapy with a doctor who specialized in suicide prevention. He treated me as if alcoholism was my only problem.

I stopped drinking and went to AA, but I still would get very depressed from time to time when I was sober. Sometimes when I fell off the wagon, I would be awake and alert around the clock no matter how much I drank. From notes I made years ago when I remembered this time better, I rarely drank when Maura and I were raising our family. But when I drank, I drank. I would go to strip bars sometimes, drunk or sober. Apparently I got involved with unsavory characters at the places where I would hang out once in a while. I remember one Christmas Eve when a guy from organized crime called to say I had to pay back what I owed, or else. I didn't remember owing money, but I paid him off.

I loved my job at the *Daily News*. I loved walking in the front door every day and seeing the huge globe of the world in the center of the lobby. I loved writing the editorials.

I was a good, come-home-from-work-every-day husband most of the time. But from time to time, I would drink. Then I led a double life, just as I did in Detroit and Albany. A professional writer during the day and a bar crawling drunk in the evening and early morning. I drank to feel better when I was depressed. Or I drank to make the good times last longer, to stoke the feeling that I was on top of the world. After a year or so Maura got pregnant. Bringing a new life into the world was about to become the most exciting and rewarding experience of my life.

I was there when Mark was born. The nurse wrapped him in a cloth and handed him to me. I was the first person to hold Mark when he came into this world.

We put a crib for Mark in a corner of our dining area. Maura left her job at the UN to stay home with our baby son. We took Mark with us whenever we could. I would strap him on my back or we would push him in the stroller.

Sometimes Maura would bring him to the lobby of the *News* building where they would wait for me to get off work. Even though he may have been too small to understand what was going on, we would take him to the Central Park Zoo and for long rides in his stroller in Central Park.

Our one-bedroom apartment was getting cramped. We needed more room for Mark. The *Daily News* paid enough for us to live on, but not enough for us to rent or buy a larger apartment. As much as we loved living in Manhattan, we moved to a small stucco house in Bayside, Queens. Now Mark could have his own bedroom and a back yard to play in with Sunshine, and Manhattan was only a short bus and subway ride away.

Emma lived next door to us and was a babysitter for Mark as much as we needed her, and they loved each other. Having such a wonderful sitter for Mark allowed us the opportunity to socialize some in Manhattan.

I was writing more editorials on health care, including a careful look at local hospitals.

The New York Health and Hospital Corporation was created in 1969 to manage the city's massive municipal hospital system.

Bellevue hospital, the best-known municipal hospital for its emergency and psychiatric care, actually started in 1736 as an infirmary for contagious diseases. A study in 1825 found filthy conditions, serious neglect of patients and positions filled by political appointments. Despite its problems, Bellevue had quite a medical history.

The medical school opened there in 1861 and a nursing school in 1873. By 1870, Bellevue had 1,200 beds. It conducted the first cesarean section in 1867 and had the first hospital-based ambulance service in 1869.

It opened the first children's clinic in 1874 and the first emergency pavilion in 1876. By 1884 it opened the first pathology and bacteriological laboratory and performed the first in-hospital appendectomy in 1887. It also opened the first ambulatory cardiac unit in 1911.

Farther north, Metropolitan and Harlem hospitals were opened in the 1870s. King's County Hospital was founded in Brooklyn in 1831. Lincoln Medical Center was the first municipal hospital in the Bronx. It opened in 1902. Queens's first municipal hospital, Elmhurst Hospital Center, opened in 1832.

By 1980 the Health and Hospitals Corporation (HHC) managed eleven acute care hospitals in all five boroughs of New York City, three large nursing homes, and scores of community clinics as well as the city's Emergency Medical Service. This massive system with more than 50,000 employees and a budget of nearly $3 billion in 1980 offered free health care to all who couldn't afford to pay for it.

It was a huge drain of city resources. With the advent of Medicare and Medicaid, the system relied less on city funds but still had huge numbers of uninsured as those with government insurance could go to private hospitals.

HHC was full of political patronage, something that has plagued municipal hospitals for centuries. It had quality of care issues, especially in the hospitals not affiliated with major medical schools. Its board of directors was made up of political appointees and some health care executives.

I wrote a series of editorials about HHC and its historic problems and drain on the city budget.

Richard Berman was in charge of the state agency that monitored hospitals. He took a keen interest in HHC. The HHC president's job was a revolving door. Four consecutive presidents resigned in the 1970s.

With Mayor Ed Koch's blessing, Deputy Mayor Bobby Wagner and Berman set out to put together a whole new management team for HHC. This certainly wasn't the first time HHC management was replaced over quality-of-care and financial-management issues.

The next new president was to be Dr. Abe Kauvar, who was credited with turning the Denver public hospital system into a fiscally sound enterprise offering high-quality care. Denver's system was described as a model for the entire country. Wagner and Koch convinced Kauvar to move to New York City to take on the municipal hospital system with its history of centuries of political patronage, quality-of-care, and crucial financial issues. I wrote several editorials encouraging the city and state to keep up their efforts to improve management of the largest non-federal health system in the world.

They brought in Kauvar and a very capable young female doctor to monitor quality-of-health issues. I think Berman or Wagner asked for O'Neill's permission first, and then they asked me to join the new team at HHC. I would be Vice President of

Public Affairs. I would be responsible for media relations and lobbying state and federal officials.

Every hospital had its own community board, and I was to interface with them and manage their activities.

Finally, I would be responsible for preparing for the board of directors meetings. I would have a pretty good staff with people assigned to each of my areas of responsibility. The best part was that the job paid $60,000 a year, which was very good money in 1980 for someone my age.

It would be my first management job where I supervised people whose work would determine my reputation.

My career in health care started with a public relations nightmare. Kauvar was talking to a community group trying to tell them he had no hidden agendas. "I don't have a ni*** in the woodpile," he said. You could hear the dead silence in the room. Did he just say what I thought he said? His audience was about 70 percent African-American.

Talk about a public relations challenge. How could I defend a person who used one of the most vile words in the English language in public?

I would say he was an older man from a different generation and a different part of the country. He meant no harm. He apologized. I said what I could to help quiet the storm, but I was personally appalled by Kauvar's remark.

The mayor sent him a note telling him he was a "good man" and to stick with his new responsibilities. The prospect of actually reforming the city's massive municipal hospital system was well worth a misstatement, no matter how offensive it was.

A young man from the mayor's office, Victor Botnick, may have been closer to Koch than anyone else in city government. Koch assigned him to look after HHC.

Kauvar didn't last long. Although it didn't help him, he didn't leave just because of the remark. It was obvious from the beginning that he was in way over his head. He was a nice man with good intentions, but he was unable to navigate the always stormy seas at HHC.

Kauvar was another one of so many medical professionals who tried to improve HHC hospitals and failed. But who could run HHC well? Koch turned to perhaps the toughest and smartest official in his government, Stanley Brezenoff, who ran the city's entitlement programs such as welfare, food stamps, and Medicaid. Botnick stayed and watched.

My job at HHC was a real pressure cooker. I had to learn the politics of every borough. I had to learn all the complex issues with state and federal agencies that monitored hospitals like ours. I had to deal with all the hospitals' community boards.

Many of their members were very well connected politically and had their own relationships with city hall. I had to deal with what I called the three B's—Botnick, Brezenoff, and Carlota Brantley, Brezenoff's top aide. They could be very difficult to please, but for the most part, they were fair.

Some of the hospitals had relationships with major medical schools that supplied their municipal counterparts with interns and residents making hospitals like Bellevue teaching hospitals. There always seemed to be public complaints from the medical schools or the municipal hospitals. The hospitals criticized the schools saying they were selling the municipal hospitals short by giving them little else than the interns and residents.

The medical schools would complain that the municipal hospitals didn't do enough for their young doctors. It seemed the only positive headlines we would get from time to time would be stories about the emergency medical service saving lives. Brezenoff was well-liked by the media, and that made my job a little easier.

Maura became pregnant with Marie while I worked at HHC. Botnick got the officers of HHC company cars. They were small blue four-cylinder vehicles. The rationale was that we had to go to the hospitals at all times day and night. The best part of these cars was they came equipped with a flashing red light and sirens.

When it was time to take Maura to the hospital to have Marie, I took the HHC car. We got stuck in traffic on a bridge into the city. Finally a good opportunity to use the red lights and siren. With the siren screaming I weaved in and out of traffic making the car jump hard from one side to the other. Maura got very nervous and the sudden movements of the car didn't help either.

She finally started screaming for me to stop. Later she told me she felt like she was going to have the baby in the front seat of the official city car.

My book was dead. It had been more than six years since my agent told me she was sure she could get it published. I lost track of her. I didn't even know if she was still an agent. I figured that either the book was no good or the agent was no good or both. I was really too busy to worry about it.

I had been working two jobs for the last few years. While at the *Daily News* I started writing fiery speeches about economic racism and economic opportunity for Earl Graves, founder and publisher of *Black Enterprise Magazine.* I continued writing for Earl when I came to HHC.

Mark was about two and a half years older than his sister. I loved having a great wife and two young children. But as much as I loved being a good father and husband, I still managed to get into trouble.

I had been sober for years when a young woman who worked for someone who worked with me invited me out to lunch. I did have lunch from time to time with my direct reports. So why not this young lady?

I knew something was amiss when she led me to the front door of her apartment building. She invited me in telling me she had something special just for me. I thought she had prepared some food for our lunch.

As soon as she shut the door behind her, I knew that something was up and it wasn't lunch. I got really nervous. I had been promiscuous when I was married to Judy.

I didn't want to be like that with Maura. I took the glass of wine she offered me, the first drink I had in years.

I had a couple more glasses and willingly participated in her idea of lunch. That taste of alcohol mixed with a great dose of guilt for what I had done started me on a roller coaster of drinking. I drank at bars day and night, pretending I was visiting this or that hospital.

One early morning an after-hours place I visited from time to time when I drank kicked me out for being too drunk and disruptive. I tried to get the police commissioner at home at five in the morning to tell him to raid the place. Thank God I didn't get through.

Finally, it all caught up with me, and I had to go to a hospital to detoxify. Then I went to a terrific rehab—Veritas Villa—in upstate New York. They still send me a Christmas card every year.

When I came home from the Villa I went back to work, and everyone seemed to welcome me back. No one mentioned the reason I was away for a few weeks. I did not continue the affair. I found out later she was having lunch with another man who was a big shot at HHC, but he didn't go on a bender over it like I did.

Chapter 6

Everything was getting more and more tense for me at HHC. It seemed like the three B's were more critical of me with each passing day. Managing HHC was a brutal task. Brezenoff, Botnick, and Brantley were under tremendous pressure to improve both the finances and the quality of care of the huge system. It got to the point where little my office did would please them. I didn't know whether the pressure was simply rolling downhill to my door or if I was really failing them.

I had worked there for four years, which was a long time for an HHC officer.

I also had worked at the *Daily News* for four years. That meant it was eight and a half years since I was as close to dying as you can get without dying. Despite the increasing unpleasantness of my job, my family life was really improving. I was making enough money for us to move to a better house. We found a big brick house I could afford in a nicer part of Queens called Bayside Hills.

Sunshine died and we replaced him with another great dog we called Maxi. I found out later from our regular trips to Ireland that half the dogs there are named Maxi. Tee ball was the sport of choice for children in Bayside. We liked it because every kid had an equal chance to get a hit.

Up to this point in my life I had never had to look for a job. I was always called and asked whether I would be interested in working for the governor of New York or the *New York Daily News* or HHC.

Mark was in first grade and Marie was still at home when I got the call from a headhunter. Would I be interested in working for Philip Morris Companies, Inc., the holding company that owned and managed Philip Morris USA, Philip Morris International, Miller Brewing, 7-Up, and a real estate venture in California?

Before Marlboro, Philip Morris's main product was an unfiltered cigarette called Philip Morris. Little Johnny, the bellboy, calling out, "Call for Philip Mooooris," was the company's main advertising. During that time, Philip Morris was in last place among America's tobacco companies.

Then Marlboro came on the scene. It took several years before it began to become popular and profitable. The first memorable commercial for the filtered cigarette was, "You've got a lot to like with a Marlboro, filter, flavor, flip-top box."

Then the Leo Burnett advertising agency in Chicago came up with the Marlboro man commercials in 1955, and over the years, with millions and millions spent on the cowboy, Marlboro cigarettes would become one of the most successful packaged-goods products in the world.

With the additional brands of Benson and Hedges, Virginia Slims, Merit, Parliament, and others, Philip Morris became the number one cigarette company in the world. Today Marlboro alone has more than 50 percent of the shrinking American cigarette market.

I interviewed with Andrew Pike, the director of communications for the parent Philip Morris Companies, Inc., for the job of manager, media relations. Pike said he was impressed with my *New York Daily News* experience. He also made it clear that he was looking for someone who could fill his job someday in case he was promoted.

Perhaps because its main product was becoming increasingly unpopular, Philip Morris took public relations very seriously. Its chairman at the time, George Weissman, came from a PR and advertising background. At that time Philip Morris had a very good corporate image. It was respected on Wall Street for its predictable ever-increasing earnings and stock price. It had earned a reputation as a well-run company with deep pockets that spent a considerable amount of money supporting the arts. It was a terrific company that just happened to make cigarettes.

The job I was interviewing for was to maintain and improve the corporate reputation by generating positive media coverage for the large, international company that appreciated good public relations.

Pike's job was to supervise internal communications including the company's employee newspaper called *Call News* after Johnny's famous "Call for Philip Mooooris." He also supervised external communications including media relations.

My job would be to supervise media relations by managing a few public relations agencies and consultants the company used. I would field questions from the media and prepare executives for media interviews. I would also write press releases.

I interviewed with a few people including the company's top PR executive, Vice President Stanley Scott. Scott happened to be a good friend of Earl Graves, the publisher of *Black Enterprise Magazine*. I had been writing Graves's speeches for several years.

I don't know if it was Graves's endorsement that did it, but I won the job offer over several other candidates. I started the new job in January of 1984.

It was back to the bus and subway to get from my home in Queens to the Philip Morris building at 120 Park. Working there was totally different than HHC. Criticism was direct but gentle. Praise for a job well done could be generous. Because I was a spokesperson for the company and because I handled interviews with top executives, I had some exposure with senior management. Many large corporations treated public relations as a troublesome and unwelcome function they had to tolerate. Philip Morris Companies, Inc., for the most part, appreciated the function.

Each of the operating companies also had a person in charge of public relations, including media relations. So I had to work with my counterparts in Philip Morris USA, and Philip Morris International. Both cigarette companies were headquartered in the Philip Morris building at 120 Park in New York where I worked. Domestic cigarettes were made in Richmond Virginia where the company held its annual meeting each year.

Miller beer was located in Milwaukee, Wisconsin. And 7 Up's headquarters were located in St. Louis, Missouri.

My job involved some travel to plants and business offices. I also traveled to locations where Philip Morris sponsored art exhibits that were opened to the press and public.

Coverage in the minority press was important to us. We had a consultant to work with the black press and another consultant to work with the Hispanic press. Both groups were mainly composed of publishers of weekly newspapers. Each group had an association we supported by sponsoring some of their events.

I ended up liking my job at Philip Morris almost as much as I enjoyed working at newspapers. At a newspaper you were judged by your copy, by the quality of the articles or editorials you wrote. At Philip Morris you were also judged by the quality of your work and the results of that work. Like everywhere else, corporate politics existed, but it was mild compared to HHC. My experience at Philip Morris demonstrated a corporate culture that rewarded high quality, results driven work with pay and promotions with a minimum of corporate politics. My job at Philip Morris was very much a people job. My success depended on my ability to get along with a wide variety of people inside and outside of the company.

Although it kept me away from my family for days at a time, for the most part, I enjoyed the corporate travel. Sometimes I traveled alone. Often I traveled with others in the company. We stayed in the best hotels and ate in the best restaurants. We worked hard and relaxed hard.

But in all of the nine years I would work for Philip Morris, I never took a drink. I smoked marijuana occasionally, but I didn't drink. Looking back, I was probably self-medicating with marijuana like I self-medicated with alcohol.

It made me feel better when I was sad and calmed me down when I was flying high.

At this time of my life, I still had mood swings from noticeable depressions to mild, euphoric highs called hypomanias. Over the years I had learned to manage these symptoms, to hide them from others. I didn't realize at the time that I had a mental illness that would have its way with me in years to come.

Things were very good at home and at work and that helped keep the symptoms more manageable. Mania in milder forms can be an asset at work. It brings faster and more accurate thinking. Mild mania can breed success. It can foster genius. But I hate to think any success I may have achieved in my career was due to a mental illness.

I remember setting up a series of senior management interviews with *Fortune Magazine* that resulted in Philip Morris Companies, Inc., being named second most admired company in America.

I was thirty-eight years old. I still weighed a trim 185. Some women I worked with from outside agencies seemed interested in more than just working with me. It didn't take too long for me to become promiscuous again.

Philip Morris sponsored the Virginia Slims tennis tournaments each year. Billy Jean King was the top women's tennis player at the time, and she helped promote the Virginia Slims tournament, which she won most of the time.

I invited reporters and editors from all types of media to come to watch the tennis. We would make sure they had enough to eat and drink. We asked for nothing in return. It was just another way Philip Morris courted the media.

I was having an affair with a woman who worked at a public relations agency that we used to help us invite and entertain the press at the Virginia Slims tennis tournament.

Instead of going to the tennis, we checked into a nearby hotel and watched the tennis on TV. When it was about over, we rushed back to the reception as if we had been there the entire time.

I made the serious mistake of leaving the receipt from the hotel in my pocket. All of my work expenses were put on a company credit card. This receipt was on my personal credit card, and it was for renting a hotel room when I was in town. Maura found the receipt and realized what it was right away. She was devastated. Her first reaction was, "What's wrong with me?" After that came the totally justified Irish temper. We went for counseling, and I stopped seeing the other woman. I think I felt as bad as Maura did over the selfish behavior. I felt terrible. I wanted to be a good father and husband. I wanted to be a man who put his family first all of the time. Maura and I had a decent sex life. We had the precious treasure of love and sex together. But, no matter how much affection and sex there was in my marriage, I always felt emotionally and sexually unsatisfied. I did not realize that my insatiable emotional and sexual needs were a specific symptom of my manic depression. Years later when I would be medicated for bipolar disorder, my sexual wanderings totally stopped.

Despite the problems in my personal life, I must have been doing very well at work.

One day Scott called me to his office. I wondered what mistake I must have made. He told me Pike was leaving the company and I was appointed to his job, Director of Corporate Communications.

I was to work closely with the tobacco, beer, and soft drink businesses in managing all internal and external communications for the parent company. I was responsible for preparing speeches for the chairman and other senior executives. I managed several people. It was the most responsibility I had so far in my career. It was the big leagues compared to HHC.

Now I really enjoyed coming to work each day. In addition to the increased responsibility, I now had privileges in the executive dining room on the top floor. When I flew on business trips, I went first class. I began to feel important.

I had smoked ever since I was a senior in high school. You

could smoke when you were a senior, so why be a senior if you didn't smoke?

At Philip Morris each employee received a carton of cigarettes a week whether they smoked or not. You could smoke anywhere. But this was the mid-eighties when you could still smoke in airplanes.

I believed the company's positions on smoking and health. Cigarettes could be habit forming, but they were not physically addictive. There were studies that showed smoking could cause cancer, but many people who never smoked battled lung cancer.

At least that's what I remember about the company's position on those issues at that time. Philip Morris USA, our domestic cigarette company, developed a program that tried to organize smokers politically so they could vote against politicians who were trying to get smoking restrictions passed into law. A large percentage of Americans still smoked. If you could organize just a fraction of them to be a political force, you might be able to stop or at least slow down the rapid growth of the anti-smoking movement.

Although they were able to put together a small political movement of sorts, the main thing learned from that campaign was that a large percentage of smokers felt guilty or uneasy about their habit and did not want to get politically involved with smoking issues.

They developed another campaign that advertised smoking as a "freedom of choice." Today Philip Morris funds programs to help people stop smoking.

As director of corporate communications, I was invited to give speeches on my own to different media organizations. I had my own freelance speechwriter. Of course I would rewrite large parts of what he wrote. I prepared speeches for the chairman.

The company had a policy that the chairman had to retire when he turned 65. Weissman retired and was replaced by Hamish Maxwell, who had been president of Philip Morris International. I was promoted when Maxwell was chairman.

For a few years there was a buzz in the media about how

cigarette companies would lose product liability cases and have to pay huge unfavorable judgments. The case the plaintiff's bar decided to put on first was the Cipollone case.

According to the attorneys who saw hundreds of millions of dollars in their future from tobacco product liability suits, the Cipollone case was their best shot. The suit was filed in 1983 blaming cigarette companies for Rose Cipollone's cancer. She died in 1984 and her husband, Antonio, continued the case. The story-line in the media was that the Cipollone case could be the beginning of the end of the cigarette industry.

The Cipollone case was the flagship of all of the product liability cases in the pipeline.

The cigarette companies were charged with fraud, conspiracy and defective product design. The basic argument was the cigarette companies conspired to mislead the public on smoking and health issues. Therefore, they were responsible for Rose's death.

The trial was a very big deal with the media. The *New York Times*, *Wall Street Journal*, Associated Press, and other national media were there to cover the trial in person.

I don't know who made the decision, perhaps it was Maxwell himself, but I was drafted to handle the press covering the trial. Part of the job was to call attention to our witnesses' testimony. We hired a very good public relations agency to help me.

The trial began in federal court in Newark, New Jersey, on February 1, 1988 before Judge Sarokin. The plaintiffs put on their expert witnesses for the first ten weeks of the trial. The tobacco industry took six weeks to put its case before the jury.

A car and driver would pick me up at my home in Queens and drive me back and forth to the New Jersey courthouse every day.

Most of my time was spent in the courtroom watching the trial. During breaks we would talk to reporters making sure they understood our side of the story. At the end of each day we made an attorney available to answer any questions they might have.

On the way home one night, my driver asked if I minded if he smoked a joint while he was driving me. Instead of firing him, I asked him for some to smoke myself. I didn't get too stoned.

When I arrived home, Maura couldn't tell I had been smoking the stuff.

I was always clear-headed in the mornings. I had to leave my house by 7:15 a.m. in order to get to the court before it opened. We had rented an office across the street from the courthouse where the attorneys would meet to prepare for the day's testimony.

I would be briefed then on what to expect that day so we could decide how to handle questions that were sure to come from the media in attendance. We prepared press releases when our witnesses made strong points to underscore our side of the story.

It is a tragedy that Rose Cipollone died of cancer. But she smoked of her own free will. She was responsible for her decision to smoke.

She must have been aware of the claims that smoking could cause cancer, and she decided to smoke anyway.

Speaking of smoking, I started to smoke marijuana more often on my way home in the evenings. The trial went on for four months. Some days created headlines, some didn't. Of course the plaintiffs received more coverage of their witnesses than we did of ours.

I found out later that one of the reasons I got the assignment to work at the Cipollone trial was that others who could have done the job were afraid they would be blamed when bad publicity came from the trial.

I was grateful for the assignment. I saw the opportunity as a challenge. Maxwell was brilliant and fair. I didn't worry about the days when the other side won the headlines for their side of the story. I just tried my best to get our side of the story in the coverage.

We waited on pins and needles during the five days the jury was in deliberations.

The jury finally reached its verdict on June 13, 1988. The cigarette companies were found not liable for Rose Cipollone's death. Philip Morris was exonerated of every charge.

But the jury did find Liggett Group, Inc., guilty of a relatively minor charge and awarded $400,000 to Mr. Cipollone.

The media coverage could have gone two ways—the cigarette companies were found not guilty of all the major charges. Or the first trial produced the first award against the industry. This was the beginning of the end of America's cigarette industry.

My challenge was to get our side of the story in the initial coverage of the verdict.

Money wasn't a problem. We set up two makeshift TV studios, each with the capacity by satellite to directly broadcast our attorneys giving our side of the story in time for the late evening news.

The system had the capacity for two-way communications so the anchors could ask the attorneys questions live on the air. With two satellite feeds going full blast, we were able to broadcast the fact that the cigarette companies were found not guilty of all the major charges to just about every major TV market. There also were radio feeds to news stations. And we put out a press release for the print media and arranged interviews with the senior attorneys.

Our side of the story prevailed in the media coverage. The jury found Philip Morris and the other companies not guilty of all the important charges. Some reporters called attention to the fact that the $400,000 reward on the minor charge against the smallest company was just a fraction of what the plaintiff's attorneys spent in prosecuting the case. It was the first and last good news on the cigarette product liability front. At the end of that day, the stock price held up. In the next year, the number of product liability cases against the industry actually decreased significantly.

Three of the attorneys from Shook, Hardy and Bacon, the firm that represented Philip Morris in the Cipollone case, went on to become top corporate officers of Philip Morris Companies, Inc.

Since Cipollone, American tobacco companies have had to pay many billions as a result of losing product liability cases.

Today the price of cigarettes in my neighborhood approaches $10 a pack, the result of the companies charging more to pay for the product liability costs. But the biggest reason for the dramatic increase was local government raising taxes so much until they became 60 to 80 percent of the cost of buying cigarettes. I quit smoking a few years ago with the help of a nicotine patch. Smoking was costing me nearly as much as car payments.

Maxwell saw the handwriting on the wall for the future of the cigarette business, and with the approval of the board of directors he began to spend the companies' considerable cash and credit to build a food business. Philip Morris should be able to manage a food business. After all the food business produced packaged goods that were sold with creative national advertising campaigns.

Philip Morris acquired General Foods in 1985 for $5.6 billion. General Foods was one of the largest food companies in the world. Some of its major brands were Maxwell House coffee, Jell-O, Oscar Mayer meats, and Post cereals. For its first two years as a Philip Morris company, General Foods didn't post much of a profit. Instead of backing off the food business, Philip Morris bought Kraft Foods in 1988 for $12.9 billion.

Being on the winning side of a hostile corporate takeover was intoxicating. Working with the media was a lot more exciting than usual. A hostile takeover attempt is the closest thing to war in the business world. It is the ultimate competition. No company wants to lose a hostile takeover battle.

Both General Foods and Kraft tried to escape Philip Morris's bid to buy them by recapitalizing and taking their stock price higher than Philip Morris's original bid.

Then the huge tobacco company just reached into its deep pockets to sweeten its bid beyond the stock price either food company could raise on their own.

We stayed up around the clock during the battles feeding the media information about our intentions for the food business.

With General Foods our entry into the food business was a natural path of growth for the consumer products giant that managed tobacco, beer, and soft drink companies. With the acquisition of Kraft, we would merge Kraft and General Foods into the nation's largest and, hopefully, most profitable food company. In my opinion getting into the food business in such a big way was a wise and prudent investment of the mountains of cash generated by the cigarette business.

Both food companies had excellent, wholesome, family-orientated images that went along with their products. How were they ever going to be able to accept being owned by the biggest bad tobacco company?

It turns out I would have a lot to do with the relationship between Philip Morris Companies, Inc., and its food business. Then the food business was called Kraft General Foods, and Maxwell asked me to be the first executive from Philip Morris to move to suburban Chicago where Kraft's offices were located. I became Senior Vice President of Corporate Affairs for the nation's largest food company.

Chapter 7

I packed a suitcase and immediately headed to Glenview, Illinois, the suburb of Chicago where Kraft's headquarters were located. I was the first Philip Morris executive to arrive at Kraft, and I was carefully welcomed to the food business. I could feel the bright focused light of hundreds of eyes looking my way, wondering just what kind of a person could work for a cigarette company, wondering if I could give them a clue of what life would be like under Philip Morris's rule.

Philip Morris Companies, Inc., now was the world's largest tobacco company, the nation's largest food company, America's second-largest brewery, and third-largest soft drink company.

My most immediate challenges involved not only internal communications between Philip Morris and its newly acquired food business but also communications between Kraft and General Foods. Philip Morris had acquired General Foods two years before Kraft. The external and internal communications had to focus on merging General Foods and Kraft into one company in the Philip Morris family. In the beginning the internal communications aimed at employees of both food companies were the most critical challenge I faced. The new company was to be called Kraft General Foods (KGF) and it was to be managed by the Kraft team in Glenview, Illinois. Michael Miles, the CEO of Kraft, would now be the CEO of the combined companies. Miles was one of the smartest people I had ever met. But he didn't much care for public relations.

I had to learn the food business while supervising communications aimed at employees and the media, explaining why the merger of the two food giants under the Philip Morris umbrella was a good deal for everyone, especially consumers and shareholders.

At first I stayed in a nearby hotel. A car and driver would pick me up each morning and bring me back when the day was done, no matter how late I worked. Kraft took care of everything. They flew my family from New York and put us up in a company apartment while we looked for a house.

I had picked out a house not too far from where most of Kraft's top management lived. But it was too near a busy intersection for Maura. Kraft's real estate experts finally showed us a house we liked in a quiet neighborhood of large homes on the east side of Barrington. It was a suitable home for a senior vice president and his family. It was much larger than our New York City house, and the two-acre lot was on the edge of a small lake. I think Kraft paid part of the down payment. I was so thrilled with my new job and the tremendous challenges I faced, I didn't pay enough attention to how the move affected my wife and children, especially my son, Mark.

It had been only six years since I was hired as a manager for media relations. Now I was a senior vice president. Instead of giving presentations, I reviewed them as a member of a select few in senior management called the Operating Committee.

I learned the food business, category by category, brand by brand, marketing campaign by marketing campaign. Kraft and General Foods were divided up into seven companies. The Operating Committee was in charge of all of them.

My specific responsibilities included internal communications between the employees of the seven operating companies and KGF's management, as well as communications about KGF to the rest of the Philip Morris world. I also was the president of the Kraft Foundation which gave out millions of dollars to worthy organizations each year.

I was also in charge of a wide variety of external communications. Our office provided speeches to senior management. My staff fielded questions from media all over the world. We pushed favorable information about our food brands and the businesses that produced and sold them. We were involved in business, food safety, and nutritional issues. In our communications we followed food from the farm to the dinner plate. We were involved with the company's larger product publicity campaigns. For example, my office worked hard on the introduction of Kraft's first fat-free products. Kraft had a large exhibit in Disney World in Florida called "The Land." that fell under my office's jurisdiction.

We had contracts with large and small public relations agencies for our publicity campaigns. With the input of my staff, an important function of my office was to choose which public relations agencies would handle our various publicity needs.

My career was defined by the excellent work of those I supervised on my immediate staff as well as consultants and members of public relations agencies.

We worked on a wide variety of projects from the introduction of new products to campaigns to introduce the new KGF to critical audiences.

In addition to my duties at KGF, I was involved in a few outside organizations. I served on the board of directors of the Gateway Foundation and the International Food Informational Council. I was a trustee of the National 4-H Council and a member of the Conference Board's Council of Corporate Communications Executives.

Meanwhile, the Ricke family, Tom, Maura, and their children Mark and Marie were trying hard to get accustomed to their new house, neighborhood, and schools.

Mark was in fifth grade and Marie was in second grade when we moved to Illinois. They both hated leaving their friends in New York. Mark had an especially hard time adapting to his new school. He found the other students very cold, and it took him quite some time to make new friends. It wasn't a cakewalk for Marie either, but, perhaps because she was younger, adjusting to the new life in suburban Chicago seemed somewhat easier for her.

Maura found Kraft's top executives and their spouses much less friendly than the Philip Morris people we left behind. She told me Kraft's top people were "less open and less caring."

I was so busy and preoccupied with work, Maura must have felt alone in caring for our children. Mark played hockey in the evenings. Marie played soccer during the afternoon and on some weekends. She was also in the Barrington Children's Choir. I did my best to attend Mark and Marie's events.

I attended hockey and soccer games, but not all of them. I traveled quite frequently and, when I was home, my business became part of the fabric of our family life.

Golf was part of the corporate culture at Kraft. When the Operating Committee traveled we would often bring our clubs on the corporate jets and find time to play eighteen holes.

Kraft paid for my membership in a country club. I wasn't a very good golfer, but I did enjoy walking down the fairways looking for my ball on weekends, weather permitting,

I would invite members of my staff or men I did business with to play golf with me. Some weekends we would golf at my club. Other weekends I would be invited to golf at a business associate's club.

I bought a set of clubs for Maura and Mark and urged them to take lessons. Maura tried it and didn't like it too much. I didn't realize how much Mark hated it because he pretended to like it to please me.

From time to time we would bring friends and/or neighbors to dine at the club with us.

The Kraft Foundation supported local cultural organizations, and the company bought season tickets for local sporting events. Senior management would take turns using the tickets. So we attended the Lyric Opera and outdoor concerts at Ravinia. We had great tickets for Bulls games so I was able to take Mark to watch Michael Jordan in his prime.

Disney rolled out the red carpet for us when I brought my family to Disney World where KGF had an exhibit that my department managed.

When I look back on it all now, we lived as American corporate royalty. First of all, we were paid very well and had bonuses and stock options as part of our compensation.

I would fly first class. And I would use a corporate jet if I was taking some of my staff with me. I had a company car, a Lincoln, and I drove back and forth to work each day. I had a company credit card and used it to cover the expenses I incurred from my work, and, since much of my time was spent working, I used the card a lot.

We could afford to do nearly anything we wanted to. Almost every year we would go to Ireland to visit Maura's family. Yes, we lived quite well.

Other members of the operating committee had been senior management for years and years, and they seemed to take it all for granted, but I kept pinching myself to make sure this life wasn't a dream. In all of my years in offices, I had some challenging and interesting work, but I never dreamed I would be a corporate officer, especially a member of senior management in a company that was so large and made so many brands that were part of everyday life in more than 140 countries. Kraft has hundreds of brands in hundreds of millions of households—some say a billion—around the world. Today nine of those brands each generate more than $1 billion a year in sales. Another fifty brands have sales of more than $100 million. Eighty percent of Kraft products are number one in their categories. Fifty percent have market shares twice their nearest competitor. At this writing Kraft has 100,000 employees in food processing plants and offices around the world. The nation's largest food company had $44 billion in annual sales, with $9.7 billion in European sales and $8.2 billion in sales in developing nations.

Philip Morris Companies, Inc., built today's Kraft.

In addition to acquiring General Foods and Kraft it purchased RJR Nabisco for $19.2 billion in 2000. Think Oreo cookies and Ritz crackers.

At first I felt inadequate. I feared I might be in way over my head. I wasn't paid to write. I wasn't paid to handle the day-to-day questions from the press. I wasn't paid to manage the daily activities of the Kraft foundation.

I had capable staff people to run the day-to-day operations. I was paid for my experienced judgment. My job was to be a leader, to supervise my talented staff, to make them feel good for their hard work. I didn't believe in raising my voice or belittling my staff when they made mistakes. At Philip Morris I had developed a loyal staff that trusted my opinions on most issues. I also wanted them to feel comfortable telling me when they disagreed with me. I tried to build the same feelings of loyalty and trust at KGF but found it more difficult.

Philip Morris tried harder than Kraft to promote its corporate reputation because of the growing public disdain for it is main product. Kraft and General Foods had wholesome reputations for wholesome food products that could be found in just about every American household. I wanted to somehow have the food business's excellent reputation rub off on its tobacco parent. My KGF staff were not used to having a parent company in charge, especially a parent company that was the international champion in making and selling products that could kill people.

The most interesting project I worked on at KGF involved the first President George Bush. He had set up a Points of Light Foundation to encourage volunteerism in America. A married couple who ran a small PR agency in Washington, DC, came to me to try to persuade me to use the Kraft Foundation to support the President's Points of Light initiative with a program the Bush administration would really like.

One of the PR firm's other clients was Mike Love of the Beach Boys. He was also interested in getting involved with the Points of Light program.

I made a few trips to Washington, DC, during this time. I

would meet with the PR firm to go over ideas for Points of Light, and I would meet with some elected officials from Illinois. As chairman of Kraft's PAC I was welcome in political circles.

On one of my visits, I went to the White House to meet the young man in charge of the Points of Light program. One thing led to another and before I knew it I was walking into the Oval Office to meet with the President. Even though we had not agreed on exactly what the Kraft Foundation would do for the Points of Light program, the President thanked me for the interest and told me he was confident the effort would be a plus for Kraft and a plus for his program. The whole thing is a blur in my memory. We sat there across from the President's desk, and I felt like I was really dreaming this time. It seemed like everything was going in slow motion. We were probably in there for about ten minutes. I was very impressed and scared I would say or do something stupid. I guess you could say I was dumbfounded by it all. And I was flying high, feeling very important and very full of myself.

Once I agreed to explore the possibility of the Kraft Foundation becoming involved in the program close to the President's heart, I started getting invited to White House events.

I have pictures of Maura and me with George and Barbara Bush. I was wearing a tuxedo in one of the pictures. We had attended an official state dinner at the White House. I have another picture from a White House event of President Bush and me shaking hands. In that picture I was wearing a dark blue suit with a red tie.

After a day's work was over during a couple of my trips to Washington, DC, the head of the PR agency and I would visit some of the popular night spots. He would hire a limo to take us around.

One night we were at a club where women were singing and dancing on a stage. I couldn't take my eyes off a beautiful young brunette dancing on the right side of the stage. I walked up to the stage and told the woman I had a limo waiting outside and if she came down from the stage immediately she could join us for the rest of the evening. After she ran backstage to change her clothes, she walked over to where I were sitting and we took off together to paint the town. On some nights my brain would speed so fast I couldn't sleep. This was one of those nights. At least I had some company in the early hours of the morning.

After a year or so I began to become more confident in my work. I was able to put together a reasonable budget and get it approved. I was able to give pretty good speeches to outside audiences. I often served as a spokesperson for the company. And I started to speak up a little to give my opinions to other members of the Operating Committee.

We acquired a European coffee and chocolate company, and we began to travel some for meetings in Europe. I remember I came home from Germany once with colorful pieces of the Berlin Wall to give to my children.

I also remember a meeting of Philip Morris's top communications executives we held at a resort in the Swiss Alps.

In the retelling of it, this part of my past life seems pretty glamorous. But all the perks, all of the company-paid goodies were designed for one purpose: to keep us working, to keep us thinking of work all of the time. And like good corporate executives we did. Work was like a religion that consumed every waking hour. It was never further away than a beeper or one of those original cell phones that felt like bricks.

Mark started to have some serious problems at school, and the school counselor suggested we send him to a psychologist who specialized in treating young teens.

After a while, Dr. Ruth Francis suggested we have a family session. It took more than a month to do it because of my travel schedule for work. We'd set a time and date and then would have to cancel it because I wasn't at home.

Every day when I awoke, I had to pinch myself to see if my life was really true. I lived in a beautiful house with a wife I adored and two terrific children. I had a job I never thought I would have, not in my wildest dreams. With all of this, I still got depressed at times, times when it would be hard for me to climb out of bed in the morning no matter what wonders the day had in store for me.

When life was like that, it was all I could do to get through the motions of a day. But I did get through the days not knowing how my moods affected relationships at work or at home.

We finally came up with an idea for the President's Points of Light foundation. We would prepare excellent materials on volunteerism and send them to every high school in America with instructions for copying them for students. It would cost more than $1 million but I felt it would be worth it. Not only would it give us—and I include Philip Morris in us—a warm and fuzzy feeling in the White House, it would put the wholesome Kraft brand behind the President's program for volunteerism in millions of homes. We set up a separate foundation for the project called "Star Serve." Mike Love of the Beach Boys promised to get some of his celebrity friends to join our effort. The White House was so pleased with Star Serve it held a special event with national press coverage to announce Points of Light programs, including ours.

Mike Love and what was left of the Beach Boys played some songs. It was an event that was a corporate public relations dream. The President publicly thanked Kraft and Philip Morris for our program. Kraft's CEO Mike Miles smiled and shook the President's hand after he said a few words. So we had a very special event which had the President praising a private company in front of the national press corps.

Kraft built a new headquarters building in Northfield and I got to choose my new furniture for my new office. One day not too long after we moved, I got a surprise visit from Philip Morris Companies CEO Hamish Maxwell. He was approaching his sixty-fifth birthday and his mandatory retirement. He was in Northfield interviewing KGF's senior management asking us our opinion on who should succeed him.

There were two obvious candidates. One was Miles. The other was Geoff Bible who had been President of Philip Morris International until Maxwell sent him to be President of Kraft where he would learn the food business. I reported directly to Bible after he arrived. Miles was named chairman and CEO of Philip Morris Companies, Inc., after Maxwell retired.

Late in 1992 the Ricke family went to Washington, DC, for their vacation. We were in the process of seeing all of the sights including a tour of the White House when I received an urgent call from Kraft headquarters. There was an emergency, and I needed to come back right away. I told the head of Kraft's HR department that I was on vacation with my family and whatever it was could surely wait a few days until we came home. He insisted I come back right away.

The whole thing must have taken a few phone calls because my family remembers how upset I was during the calls. I left Maura and the children in Washington while I flew back to Northfield. I was driven straight from the airport to corporate headquarters where the VP of Human Resources was waiting for me. My worst fear was about to be realized.

Someone in the company had made a serious charge about me. I couldn't know who made the charges. I was given a choice. Leave the company with a substantial amount of money from the sale of my Philip Morris stock options and an advance of my bonus or stay and fight the charges.

If I decided to fight the charges the battle would probably end up in court where it could generate negative media coverage for me and my family. I knew I was innocent of the accusations, but I decided not to get into a public fight about it. I decided to take the money and run, a decision I regret to this day.

Philip Morris USA began to lose multi-billion-dollar product liability cases with the rest of the US tobacco industry. Meanwhile Marlboro kept gaining market share of a declining US cigarette business. With much higher local taxes and billions in additional product liability costs the cost of a pack of cigarettes skyrocketed. Yet the profit margins of both the domestic and international cigarette business were still somewhat higher than the profit margin of the Kraft food business.

Miles became the only CEO of Philip Morris Companies, Inc. to leave before his mandatory retirement date. He was CEO of Philip Morris for only two years. Before he retired Maxwell told me he thought I was innocent of the charges that ended my career with Kraft and that the charges were "out of character" for me.

Geoff Bible became CEO of Philip Morris Companies after Miles left and he was an excellent CEO until he retired when he turned sixty-five.

In January 1995, KGF became Kraft Foods and the General Foods name was gone forever. KGF's seven operating companies became one company called Kraft Foods. The company's head-quarters stayed in Northfield, and Kraft's $16 billion international business was headquartered in Zurich, Switzerland.

In the third largest IPO in history, 280 million shares of Kraft Foods were issued in 2001. Philip Morris Companies retained 88.1 percent of Kraft's stock. In January of 2003 Philip Morris Companies, Inc., changed its name to Altria. It still owned 88 percent of Kraft, all of Philip Morris USA and all of Philip Morris International. It also owned a part of Miller Beer.

In January of 2007, Altria got out of the food business completely by giving the rest of the Kraft shares to Altria stock-holders. They got 70 percent of a Kraft share for every share of Altria stock they owned. The motives seemed to be to protect Kraft from cigarette product liability lawsuits and to increase the benefits of owning Altria stock.

In February of 2008, Warren Buffett, one of the richest people in the world known for his savvy investments in rock solid compa-nies, spent more than $4 billion for an 8 percent share of Kraft Inc. In September of 2008, Kraft became a member of the Dow Industrial Average. Buffet must have been pleased with his invest-ment in Kraft because he increased his position to 9.4 percent of the company.

Altria spun off Philip Morris International (PMI) in 2008. Now PMI has 15 percent of the world cigarette market and is growing market share substantially by selling cigarettes, especially Marlboros, in 160 countries.

As I write this, Altria is solely in the nicotine and alcohol busi-ness. It acquired a smokeless tobacco company and the fastest growing winery in the US while it maintained a percentage of

Miller Beer. I think it was a mistake for Altria to get out of the food business leaving behind a $44 billion yearly business with perhaps a billion consumers around the world including 99 percent of American households.

Kraft took away my perks immediately after I agreed to leave. They picked up my company car and cancelled my country club membership and my corporate credit cards. They eliminated my job by having my department report directly to the senior vice president of the legal department. As far as I know, the Kraft Points of Light program died as soon as I left the company.

Kraft is water way under the bridge for me today. I worked there more than twenty years ago. Immediately after I lost my job at Kraft, I fell down a bottomless hole of depression. It was worse than depressions alone; it was manic depression, a madness that would disable me for the next two decades.

Chapter 8

I walked around in an extremely sad and forlorn daze. I figured the severe depression was a normal reaction for such a profound loss. Soon I found myself living with a dangerous combination of depression and mania at the same time. It was like being high on speed while being dragged across a field of barbed wire and ground glass. Extreme energized pain and plenty of it. At the time I had no idea what was happening to me.

After a few weeks, I got a call from a prominent headhunter asking me if I would be interested in interviewing for the top public relations position in a large company located in Houston. I hated the thought of dislocating my family again just as they had settled into their new life in suburban Chicago, but I had to be able to support us, and the job sounded interesting.

I flew to Houston and stayed in a hotel near the corporate headquarters I would visit the next day. I had dinner by myself in the hotel restaurant that contained what looked like a very popular bar filled with rows of professionally dressed people having a good time after another day in the office.

I don't remember whether I had a real drink or a diet Coke. But I will never forget the pretty brunette who walked over and started a conversation with me. She said she too was visiting

Houston on a business trip. After twenty to thirty minutes of chit chat, we were suddenly talking about whether we would end up in her room or mine.

After we walked into my room, she whipped out a badge, announced she was a policewoman, and yelled to other undercover cops outside the door who put me in handcuffs and led me to a waiting patrol car. They read me my rights. I don't remember the exact wording of the charges.

It was either for agreeing to pay or actually paying money for sex with an undercover policewoman posing as a prostitute. It was probably a misdemeanor. But whatever the charges, they were taking it very seriously as they put me in jail for the rest of the night.

My appointment with the CEO of the company that was interested in me was for 10 a.m. the next day. There was no way I was going to make it. I knew I didn't agree to pay money for her services. I had never paid for sex. And I know for sure no money changed hands. I had about $80, which was still in my wallet when they took it as I was processed in the jail.

I had a very hard time believing what was happening to me. I just wanted to wake up and have the nightmare be over. Just a few months before my trip to Houston, I was attending a special event in the White House that called attention to a civic-minded program I had developed. I was flying high in corporate jets and living well at the country club. Now I was unemployed and sitting in a Texas jail wearing the same suit and tie I wore to the White House.

I was wide awake and full of frightened energy all night. I told anyone in a uniform who would listen to me that I had an important job interview in the morning.

At around 9 a.m. they let me use a phone. One of the guards gave me the number of a Houston criminal attorney. I called him, and he called Maura and told her I was in jail. She would have to wire $7,000 for his initial fees and ten percent of the bond I would soon have to pay to get out of jail. I also called the office of the CEO I was supposed to see that morning and said I must have eaten something that didn't agree with me and that I was sick to my stomach. I asked if he would see me later in the day when I hoped to feel better.

When we got to court I was arraigned, and the judge set a date for a trial and a $10,000 bond to get me out of jail. Maura called our financial advisor and had him wire the money to the attorney. I was finally free about 4 p.m. I was a mess after a night in jail.

I took a cab back to the hotel, changed and cleaned up quickly and grabbed another cab to take me to my delayed interview. His secretary let me in to see him right away. It was close to 6 p.m. We shook hands and he asked me if I was feeling better. I remember not feeling tired after missing a night's sleep. He asked me questions and we talked for about twenty minutes. He was being polite but the whole conversation seemed to be focused on what I was going to do next with my career. After a while I realized that working for his company didn't seem to be an option on the table.

I was probably paranoid, but I thought he might have found out about my arrest. At the end of the interview, he wished me well in whatever happened next in my life.

Perhaps he had already decided to hire someone else. Or it could have been that I really screwed up the interview. I'll never know. I didn't hear from him again.

Since I had no criminal record, my attorney was able to get a deal that I would plead guilty to a misdemeanor and pay a fine. He told me that to fight the charges would cost me several thousand dollars, and there was little chance I would win. It was her word against mine, and she was the law. I had to fly back to Houston a couple of weeks later to keep my court date.

I felt so ashamed for what I had done. I was not guilty of hiring a phony prostitute, but I did agree to go to my room for a sexual encounter. That wasn't against the law, but it was a serious crime in my marriage.

The double whammy of losing my job and then spending a night in a Texas jail was too much for me to handle. At the time we knew I was severely depressed, but we had no idea that I was bipolar. I was so out of it, Maura called Dr. Francis, and she agreed to see me. After one session she knew I needed lots of help. She referred me to another psychologist because she thought seeing Mark and me at the same time might be a conflict. The new psychologist strongly believed in cognitive therapy.

He tried to get me to reward myself for making positive changes in my thoughts and behavior. I'm sure that type of therapy worked with some people with behavioral disorders, but it wouldn't work for me. Although I didn't know it, I had a case of rapid cycling manic depression. It could be set off or made much worse by traumatic events, and it certainly affected my behavior, but its cause wasn't psychological.

It was caused by a physically sick brain, by faulty brain chemistry, and cognitive therapy just did not work for my damaged brain. Medication with therapy is the most effective way to treat the symptoms of manic depression.

At the time I wasn't taking medication, and I became dangerously suicidal. I did some research and discovered I'd had my life insurance policy long enough that it would pay Maura some $850,000 if I killed myself. That would be on top of the generous settlement I received from Kraft a few months earlier. If I ended my life, I would also end the horrific inner pain I was suffering, and my family would be financially set for the rest of their lives. And they deserved someone better than me, someone who would be totally faithful to Maura and a positive role model for Mark and Marie.

I became so suicidal that I had to be hospitalized in a psychiatric hospital, Linden Oaks Hospital in Naperville Illinois. This was my first very serious bout with suicide since my self-induced coma eighteen years before. Now I had fallen from corporate jets to being locked up in jail to being locked up in a psychiatric hospital to save my life.

The last time I was overwhelmed by powerful suicidal commands that seemed to overcome me suddenly was after my altercation with Judy. This time the suicidal thoughts built up in my mind gradually, becoming stronger week after week, month after month until they became psychotic orders for me to follow. I was fortunate this time to be hospitalized before I acted out the suicidal ideations.

They put me on a twenty-four hour suicide watch my first few days in the psychiatric ward.

The hospital's report on my stay there read: "The 45-year-old married patient required hospitalization because of his increased depression and suicidal ideations. . . during the three months before his hospitalization, the patient continued to show a rapidly increasing sense of despair, helplessness, and hopelessness. In addition, he showed rapid tangential and pressured thoughts, and appeared to be hypomanic as well as severely depressed.

"He appeared hyperalert and hypervigilant. The patient graduated from college with a degree in writing and had become involved in politics. He tended to focus intellectually on things but was overrun by his emotional hungers. His affect was hypomanic and sad with some agitation. His judgment was generally intact, but he was unable to control it because of rapid mood cycling and irritability.

He lacked any insight into his current situation. His strengths were his intellectual abilities, his verbal abilities, and his ability to articulate."

Dr. Martin Krause conducted the initial interview and diagnosed me as "major depression, recurrent episodic and bipolar disorder, rapid cycling."

I had been going to mental health professionals off and on for more than twenty years, and none had diagnosed me with manic depression. I could only wonder how my life would have been different if my bipolar disorder had been diagnosed in my mid-twenties when I first exhibited mental symptoms.

After some therapy in the hospital with Dr. Krause, I realized that I had been suffering milder symptoms of manic depression throughout my professional career and marriage. The milder manias could release bursts of creative thinking and constructive energy.

The more serious manias would keep me up all night with racing thoughts running around and around in my brain. When I was either too manic or too depressed, I would shut the door of my office and read work materials so I wouldn't have to interact with people. On occasion I would be so depressed I couldn't get out of bed and would have to call in sick.

The symptoms attacking me since I lost my career were even more severe. My deep despondent depression flirted with suicide and my manias were laced with psychosis. I even had a few hallucinations.

A large percentage of people with bipolar disorder use alcohol and drugs to self-medicate. They are known to go on shopping sprees regardless of whether or not they have money to pay for them. They can have dramatic hallucinations. In fact an expert on the illness told me that you could put the symptoms of manic depression and schizophrenia side by side on a blackboard and with a few exceptions they could be pretty much the same. The most powerful symptom of manic depression is suicide. From what I read, seventy percent of patients with bipolar disorder attempt suicide. Twenty percent are successful.

I spent a month recovering on my first trip to Linden Oaks. They had me take a few medications which they monitored closely. I continued to take the medication after I was released. The day after I returned home from the hospital Paul Fulmer knocked on the front door of our house. He told me he was president of a small public relations agency in downtown Chicago and was looking for someone to take his place when he retired.

Two of his biggest clients were IGA supermarkets and Sargento Cheese. He thought my experience with Kraft made me a perfect candidate for the job of executive vice president of the Seltz Seabolt agency.

I accepted the job even though I was hoping to find a position with a large company.

As I told him I could start in a few weeks, I knew that it would be very difficult for me to be successful at the new company given the state of the mental illness which still had me in its delusional grip. The suicidal voices were still alive in my head.

The urges went from medium to very strong.

Even though I tried to fight them, the suicidal ideation became so powerful I ended up in Linden Oaks a second time. It was obvious that the medications I was taking weren't working well enough to control the most dangerous symptom of my manic depression.

Dr. Krause was frustrated with the lack of success with my illness. It was the rapid cycling that made it more difficult to treat. Most bipolar patients have rather long periods of depression followed by long periods of mania. Often they have months of normality in between the dramatic ups and downs. As a rapid cycler, my dramatic mood swings could go from psychotic mania to deep depression in a month or a week or a day.

Dr. Krause referred me to a mental health practice at Rush University Medical Center that was known for its treatment of bipolar disorder. A young woman became my psychiatrist. I was self-medicating with alcohol at the time. To keep me sober she said she wouldn't treat me if I drank again. I started another period of sobriety in my life.

The suicidal ideation was still with me. Sometimes it was fairly quiet. Sometimes it grabbed me by the throat.

I began working at Seltz Seabolt after my second hospitalization at Linden Oaks. Some days I drove downtown through terrible rush hour traffic to the tall building where the public relations agency had its office. Other days I took the train. I wasn't nearly as effective there as I was at Philip Morris or Kraft. All my experience and talent seemed to have been sucked out of me.

I went through the motions and treaded water for the most part, but I was in no shape to help run the small agency. A big part of my responsibility was to attract new business. I was used to hiring public relations agencies, not getting business for them. I also was to manage the Sargento Cheese and IGA supermarket accounts.

I had some additional hospitalizations when I worked at the Chicago firm. My super active bipolar disorder made it nearly impossible for me to succeed. I still battled with suicide. The firm was located high up in the office building. I think we were forty stories up. There was a three-foot ledge you could walk on outside of the window in my office. After everyone left for the day, I would open the window and look down at the tiny cars.

I could see myself dancing on that narrow ledge. Before the hallucination could come true, I found myself back in Rush University Medical Center's psychiatric unit.

They had me on Valium among other prescriptions. The Valium made me feel better, made me feel sort of like I was drinking. I had an appointment with the CEO of Sargento Cheese. The office was located in Wisconsin not far from the Illinois border. I took an extra Valium. If one made me feel good then two would make me feel even better.

We talked for more than an hour. I told him about my experience with Kraft. I thought the meeting went quite well. When I arrived back at the office, Fulmer asked me to step into his office. He closed the door. Then he told me that after I left Sargento, the CEO called him and told him that if he ever sent Tom Ricke to Sargento again, the agency would lose his account. To this day I have no idea what I said that caused so much trouble.

I did manage to bring in some new business before I was asked to leave. I called Hamish Maxwell, the retired Philip Morris CEO, and talked to him about my failed efforts to bring in new business. He had controlling interest in a California company that made and sold a variety of vitamins. He hooked me up with the company, but I left the agency before any deal was consummated. The agency did manage to get the account after I left, and today I understand a vitamin company is one of their largest clients.

While I worked at Seltz Seabolt I was in the hospital too much. They let me go because I just wasn't around enough to do my job. I understood perfectly, and I didn't blame Fulmer or his company for getting rid of me.

I found myself in Rush's day psychiatric program. Rush was very near downtown Chicago. Some days I drove my car. I had bought a used Harley, and on other days I would navigate on it in rush hour traffic. During nice weather we would sit outside at picnic tables and work on craft projects. I felt like I was in grade school.

Mark was having his own psychiatric issues as he was seeing Dr. Francis. I still don't fully understand the reasons, but our mental health professionals decided it would be better for Mark if I didn't live at home.

At the time they told me they were doing this to save me the brutal commute every weekday. They didn't mention a word about Mark and his perception of his father.

They put me up in an apartment near the hospital in a building where there were several units set aside for psychiatric patients. I had a roommate. His name was Henry, and he was in the same psychiatric day program that I attended.

Every evening residents of a different apartment would cook for all the psychiatric boarders. I remember Henry and I always made spaghetti with sauce out of a jar.

Maura, Mark, and Marie would visit me on weekends. They would stay for a couple of hours, and their weekend presence in my life made me miss them terribly during the long weeks. I lived in the hospital apartment for about nine months. I moved back home for insurance reasons.

Maura and I had not been intimate for a long time, and our emotional abstinence hurt me more and more as the weeks and months passed by. We were in a vicious circle that would last for years to come. The sicker I got the more distant she became, and the less frequently we would have sex. We would go many months without it. The further Maura removed herself from me the sicker I got. Round and round, down and down we went with my manic depression building a steel wall between us.

I was tortured with an obsession that would eat at me for years and push me deeper and deeper in pain and psychosis. My delusion was believing Maura was having an affair. If she wasn't having any emotional or sexual experience with me, she must be satisfying those needs with someone else.

Every time she left the house for any length of time my mind would be filled with images of her with some other man. My psychiatrist and psychologist would judge the level of my mental illness by the intensity of my delusions that Maura was having an affair.

I was in and out of the inpatient psychiatric ward on a regular basis. I certainly wasn't getting any better. When I was home, I frequently stayed in bed most of the day. It was just too painful to get up. Then I would go through periods when I would be awake for days with thoughts and illusions spinning around in my brain.

I remember one gigantic spending spree. I bought myself a Rolex watch that was encrusted with small diamonds. I bought Maura a lovely mink coat. I also bought her a diamond tennis bracelet. I bought computers for Mark and Marie. And I bought another motorcycle for myself.

I had gotten rid of the Harley because the medications I took made it difficult for me to keep my balance and made my reactions very slow. This time I bought the biggest Honda they made. I did all of this shopping in less than a week.

Maura persuaded me to take the Rolex back, but she kept the fur coat. I was lucky I had enough money to pay for it all. Many bipolar victims go on sprees they cannot afford.

I was on a merry go round of different medications. I would take a combination that would seem to work. Then after some time they would seem to stop working. I would get so suicidal I would have to go back to the hospital.

Then I would be put on a different combination of medicines that would work, but only for a limited time. Then suicidal ideations would take hold of me and convince me that only death would end the horribly painful depressive side of my bipolar disorder. As the days went by, every movement, every breath seemed to cause more and more unbearable inner pain.

I moved in slow motion. I had no sense of balance. I urinated in our bed and Maura moved into another room. I stayed in bed for days at a time.

I kept writing suicide notes trying my best to explain why my death would really be a blessing. It would end my horrific pain, and it would end all the difficulties my illness caused for my family. I just had to be convincing so they would not suffer by my leaving this world.

Here is one note that I wrote: "I just can't go forward anymore. I just can't live like this anymore. They say suicide is a permanent solution to a temporary problem. My incredible pain, my agony, my very difficult uphill struggle—none of this is temporary. I have suffered with manic depression much of my adult life. It has never, ever left me alone. No matter what or how many medications I take, the illness always comes back to have its way with me.

"This is the same illness that ruined our marriage, the same illness that totally wrecked my professional life. Now it is taking my life. It has tried before and come very close. If you are reading this note, then I have finally succeeded.

"Maura, when you think of me, I want you to realize how very much I love you. Because I love you so much, our lack of affection and intimacy gives me more deep pain than I can bear."

I put the note in the glove compartment of my car. About a month after I wrote the note, I started drinking again, pouring gasoline on the fire of my manic depression. It wasn't too long before I drove to a nearby Metra station where people commuted back and forth from downtown Chicago. It was in August, and it was very hot. I brought all of my pills and a bottle of bourbon with me. I was told I parked my car so that only a parking meter partially blocked a straight shot to the train tracks.

I started to take my pills, washing them down with swigs of whiskey. I took handfuls of three or four at a time. The radio was blaring. The air conditioning was going full blast. I took the note from the glove compartment and put it on the dashboard. I kept drinking and taking pills. Finally, I must have passed out before I could drive the car to the railroad tracks. Someone saw me slumped over with the engine running and pills scattered all over the front seat where an almost empty bottle of bourbon also could be seen and called 911.

Ever since I lost my job at Kraft the suicidal thoughts had been building and building in me. They would become stronger and somewhat weaker and then stronger again. They never seemed to leave me alone. During the time when I was being tormented with compelling thoughts of my death, I was growing weaker and weaker inside. Losing my career, my marriage, and my self-esteem gave my illness the excuse it needed to finally take control of my ever-weakening inner self. Millions of people lose jobs and withstand the emotional devastation of broken marriages, but they don't even think of suicide as an option to ending their troubles.

Whatever it is about bipolar disorder that breeds suicide in so many of its victims made me much different from other people going through rough times. I welcomed my death. I really wanted to die. I didn't think of my wife and children and parents and brother and sisters and how my self-inflicted death would cause them unbearable pain. All I could think about was turning off the switch and giving in to the sweet end of my life.

This time I fell into a coma again. Then doctors told Maura that I could very well die. I came out of it in three or four days. When I awoke and realized who I was and what I had done, I was upset to still to be alive. Maura called my psychiatrist and she said she could no longer see me as a patient because I drank again.

So there was Maura with a very troubled Mark and a husband who just came out of a coma from a suicide attempt and was without a doctor to care for him.

They transferred me back to the psychiatric ward of Rush University Medical Center where I was still upset to be alive. That psychiatric unit had become my home away from home.

Dr. Michael Easton, who was with the same mental health practice at Rush, took over my case. Although my situation would get even worse in the coming years, Dr. Easton stuck with me. He is still my psychiatrist today.

Chapter 9

After five weeks I was released from the hospital. I still walked in slow motion bent over like an old man. I never made eye contact with people. I had little sense of balance. I could not ride a bicycle. I tried it twice and ended up on the pavement. I could not stand on a chair and change a light bulb. When I walked up and down the stairs I had to hold onto the handrail with both hands. I was sad and weepy. I spent much of my days in bed.

The only thing that would get me out of bed in the afternoon was the *Ricki Lake* television show. This writer who had won awards, this executive who once had worldwide responsibilities for the world's second largest food company, this person lived to watch an afternoon television show. I felt a real connection with her. I read somewhere that she lost a lot of weight. As I mentioned, I lost 110 pounds in my mid-twenties. She was my soulmate. Watching this television show and taking a shower were all I could manage those days.

Finally, two months after I awoke from my coma, I found enough energy to do something. I returned to the girlie bars and started drinking again. I felt so bad I figured a couple of drinks would make me feel better. My prescription medicine didn't seem to be working. Let those good times roll. Let the liquid magic work.

One night I stopped in two bars where I was trying to pace myself so I would not get in trouble. I had no more than four drinks. I drove from bar to bar looking for the good feelings that would take away my troubles and give me reason to live again.

Two police cars followed me on my way home. Their lights and sirens were going full blast, but I didn't hear or see them. The car stereo was turned way up. I was much higher than I should have been from a few drinks. I continued to mix my prescription medicine with alcohol.

After a few minutes I noticed the police cars and pulled to the side of the road to let them go by. I thought they must be following someone else. I came out of the fog to see a policeman with his gun drawn. They stopped me because I had a flat tire and was driving on the right rim. Sparks were flying. I didn't realize I had a flat. They pulled me out of the car and gave me a breathalyzer test, which I failed by a small margin. They charged me with driving under the influence. They put me in handcuffs and took me to the police station lockup. They had the car towed. Here I was locked up again for a few hours before Maura came to get me.

While I continued to get worse, my wife consulted with an attorney to see if she could have all of our assets put in her name alone. She also explored the possibility of having me committed to a state mental hospital.

This arrest started sixteen months of court activity. I lost my driver's license. I had to go to special classes and do some community service. Dr. Easton put me on Antabuse, a drug that makes you violently ill if you drink with it in your system. I had heard horror stories of people drinking on Antabuse. Taking it kept me sober for more than a decade.

When Mark first started seeing Dr. Francis, he told her he really admired me for being a good dad and for the success I had earned in business. Now I wasn't fully aware of it but Mark was telling Dr. Francis that he hated me for trying to kill myself.

He hated me for being so weak and so sick. Mark's life was becoming more and more troubled. After we arrived from New York, Mark started to do poorly in school. He always seemed distracted. He stopped doing any homework. He would read books that had nothing to do with his schoolwork. Sometimes he would do some homework and not hand it in.

I don't know how much Maura knew, but I was still very sick and not totally aware of what was going on with our son. He scored very high on an IQ test, but he was in serious danger of failing his courses. The highest mark he got was a C minus. His other grades were D's and D-minuses. We made excuses for him. He was going through normal growing pains. The move from his friends in New York was traumatic for him. I thought he would get over this in a short time. His grades continued to nosedive.

For eighth grade we sent him to a Lutheran school where there was a program in which students had to do their homework before they went home. Mark did a bit better there, but he still engaged in troublesome behavior that I was not aware of at the time.

He would get up in the middle of the night and ride his bike through the neighborhood. He would frequently smoke during his nighttime excursions—either cigarettes or marijuana or both. He drank alcohol a neighbor friend stole from his parents. Eventually he would try LSD.

Some of his Barrington classmates called him "pyro" because he liked to set fires. He was never caught, but he set a few fields on fire. One time when we were visiting my brother in Detroit for a family reunion, Mark took some of his cousins to a nearby field and they watched as he set it on fire. None of them told on Mark because they were afraid of what he might do to them if they turned him in.

Before he arrived at his early teen years, Mark was always a good boy. I was there in the hospital room when he was born. He was a good baby. We often wrapped him up and took him with us when we went walking in Central Park.

I was with him when he took his first steps. He was so pleased with himself. He slept through the night. He got along very well with babysitters. After Marie was born, the two little Rickes were inseparable. They each had their friends from kindergarten and grade school, but at home they were each other's best friend. They rarely fought. We felt the same way I suspect most parents feel about their offspring. Mark and Marie were the most wonderful, cutest, smartest, most lovable small children in the world.

Mark escaped trouble for egging houses in the neighborhood, but he did get in trouble for throwing stones at the Lutheran school where he attended eighth grade. He was still seeing Dr. Francis every week.

Here is a letter he wrote to his grandparents when he was in middle school shortly after he moved from New York:

Dear Grandpa and Grandma,
How are you? I am fine.
I'm sitting down writing this while blasting heavy metal on the stereo system.
Well, first things first. Sorry about not writing to you sooner but being 15 writing a note is the last thing I would want to do. My hair is past my shoulders and the school still accepts it. They say that as long as it is neat they will let me in.
I refuse to get a haircut and as soon as I leave middle school to go to high school I am going to grow it like a headbanger.
I'm learning to play the drums and I am pretty good. It's harder than most people think. You need fast hands and a lot of good reflexes.
My bunny died and that was very sad. We buried her in the back yard.
I am going to send you a tape with the recording of a poem I call Free, a story I call the trails and a story I just started to write. I plan to be a writer like my dad when I grow up.
I'm going to get a collection of short stories I wrote and send them to a publisher soon.

He started to play hockey and we encouraged him to stick with it. At this point in his young life, Mark never finished anything he started. We attended his hockey games and cheered him on.

I had attended a Jesuit high school, and it had been very good for me. I figured that a Jesuit high school would be good for Mark too. Even with his poor grades, he was accepted into the local Jesuit school because of his high IQ. It didn't hurt that his dad was a successful graduate of both Jesuit high school and college.

Mark agreed to go to summer school, and he got his long hair cut to conform to school policy. At the time he was feeling good about high school with the Jesuits. He told Dr. Francis that he was happy to go to the same kind of high school his dad attended.

However, the Jesuits were unable to guide Mark to any type of academic success. He still didn't do his homework. He didn't study for tests. He still didn't finish anything he started. He continued to sneak out in the middle of the night to smoke cigarettes and pot. It got to the point where Dr. Francis thought he should go to a psychiatric hospital. He went to Linden Oaks, the same hospital I first tried, because it had a separate unit devoted to teens that had an excellent reputation for positive results.

Maura and I were shocked and stunned when Mark was diagnosed with bipolar disorder. We hoped and prayed that he would be spared all the painful symptoms I was suffering.

We found it difficult to accept. Didn't all teens have mood swings that were normal for adolescents? In retrospect it made some sense. He was apparently self-medicating with drugs and alcohol just like his father. It took us a while to realize that he wasn't just a mixed-up teenager. He was a mentally ill teenager. Who wants to admit that about their child?

Meanwhile I continued to suffer more extreme symptoms of manic depression. I continued to see Dr. Francis myself. She was pessimistic about my future. I also continued visiting Dr. Easton on a regular basis. From time to time, I lived in the psychiatric ward at Rush University Medical Center. I felt dull and stupid.

Then I would become manic and paranoid about Maura and the people she worked with.

I truly believed they were in a conspiracy against me.

On a scale of one to ten my depression's inner pain was at least twelve. I also had hallucinations. I saw a man standing next to our neighbor's house with a gun in his hand. I called 911 and the police who arrived very quickly told me there was no one there as I was still seeing the dangerous man.

Mark had to go to Linden Oaks a second time during his freshman year. At that time, I was in Rush. Maura would drive to Naperville to visit Mark and then to downtown Chicago to visit me. Manic depression was having its way with our family.

All of this was hard on Marie too. She didn't understand why her father didn't get up every morning and go to work like all of her friends' fathers did. She was so very frustrated that there was little she could do to help her brother. As all of this was going on in the Ricke family, Marie continued to get all A's in school. She was making friends she would keep well into her thirties, but the psychiatric turmoil in her family often caused her to stay in her room and cry. And it was very hard on Maura too, who became really depressed over losing a husband and son to manic depression.

Before he was asked to leave the Jesuit high school, Mark found out about a summer hockey camp at Notre Dame in South Bend, Indiana, where my parents grew up. My parents were visiting when we drove Mark to Notre Dame. I was so happy to see him take an interest in something.

We got a call from Notre Dame that evening. Mark wanted to come home. Could we come and get him as soon as possible?

My dad and I drove back to South Bend to pick Mark up. He didn't say anything, and we left him alone. After he fell asleep in the back seat, I remember thinking three generations of Ricke men are riding in this car. Two of them have experienced the success that comes from hard work. I prayed that Mark would soon learn that too.

After his second hospitalization, Mark attended a program with other teens with mental illness where they would do school-work and take part in some sort of group therapy.

He did okay there. There was no homework. They finished their work in class.

The program was covered by health insurance. After a while, the insurance stopped paying. They had strict limits for the treatment of mental illness, limits that did not apply to any other illnesses. And they determined that Mark's bipolar disorder was a preexisting condition. When the insurance stopped its coverage, Mark ended up going to the local Barrington public high school. Times had certainly changed since my generation attended high school. I was lucky to get a night of driving the family station wagon on a date. Now students expected a gift of a car on their sixteenth birthday so they would have their own car as soon as they got their drivers licenses. Most of them did get their cars when they turned sixteen. The parking lot at Barrington High School rivaled the lots of the most affluent car dealerships in the Chicago area.

Mark still continued to see Dr. Francis every week, and he took his prescription medication for his mental illness.

At the time we could have paid for Mark's program after the insurance ran out. It was expensive, but we still had some funds from my days at Kraft.

If we had kept him in that program, he might still be with us today.

Mark and I used to stop in a restaurant on the way to his visits with Dr. Francis. One time he told me he would love a part-time job in a place like that. I later spoke to the manager and he agreed to hire Mark to wash dishes and clean up. Mark didn't work there very long. One day he took off his apron and left with some friends who were going to a concert.

Mark continued to do poorly at Barrington High School despite the special interest of a couple of teachers and a counselor. We knew he was bipolar like me, but we didn't connect the dots between his illness and his behavior. I didn't fully realize that his troubles in school were symptoms of an illness that came from my genes. We didn't fully understand that he was self-medicating with alcohol and drugs just like his father had done for decades. He also would sneak cigarettes whenever he could. He would take them from the carton I bought every week.

But was this behavior caused by mental illness? Didn't all teens have noticeable ups and downs? Didn't they experiment with drugs and drinking and cigarettes? Couldn't his failures in the classroom be caused by the normal difficulty in growing up? I knew he was diagnosed with manic depression, but I never fully understood how it affected his behavior. I guess I was hoping against hope that he would not suffer with manic depression like I did. The truth was he was still a good boy with an illness he couldn't control.

His admiration for me turned into disgust, especially after my suicide attempt. He told Dr. Francis he could not understand what was wrong with me that would cause me to want to die. He told her he hated suicide. It got to the point where if I walked into a room where he was, he would leave the room. It broke my heart.

Meanwhile he made a couple of new friends at Barrington High School. His favorite friend was a boy named Kevin who liked to ride skateboards with Mark. They also smoked pot and experimented with LSD. Mark had a couple of girlfriends. Just before he turned fifteen, he told Dr. Francis that he had his first sexual experience.

He settled on a girl named Carol. They saw each other after school each day before they got on their school buses, and they frequently visited each other's homes. They went to the movies. She seemed like a very nice girl, and we were glad Mark was seeing her.

A few months after my suicide attempt Mark said he didn't want to see Dr. Francis anymore. He was sick and tired of her "psychobabble." We agreed with Dr. Francis that we couldn't really force him to see her. We hoped he would change his mind. Then he stopped taking his medication. That scared me. Maura and I both pleaded with him to take the pills. One time I even tried to open his mouth and force the pills down his throat.

"Trust me, Dad," he would say all the time. "I know what I am doing." Mark seemed to live for the moment. He seemed totally unconcerned about his future, unconcerned even about the next day.

After going with Carol for a while, he started to do a little better in school. He still didn't do all of his homework, but he seemed to be paying more attention in class.

Meanwhile, despite all the therapy I was getting from Dr. Francis and Dr. Easton, I continued to suffer harshly with my bipolar disorder. I was still paranoid about Maura. I believed she was plotting to take our money and run away with another man. My illness still kept me chained to my bed before Ricki Lake came to me on television and Maura came home from work. I cried all the time and was suicidal.

On February 6, 1995, Mark's sixteenth birthday, Maura and I took Mark and Carol to dinner at a German restaurant on Rand Road in Lake Zurich. It was his favorite place to eat. Presents were exchanged during dessert.

I told him I always said I would give him the shirt off my back. I took my new black leather Harley Davidson jacket off and gave it to him. He loved it.

I was still very ill and flirting with suicide. I cried and cried. I still had some hallucinations. They were weird and gross and ugly. Even though they showed me impossible sights, I saw them with great clarity. They seemed very real to me.

Maura and I continued to fight over our sex life. She didn't seem at all interested in making love with me. A social worker we saw suggested I make a bath for Maura when she came home from work.

I did it and she showed interest in making love, but I couldn't get an erection. I would find out later that sexual dysfunction could be a side effect of the medicine I was taking.

At Walmart with Maura I stared at the gun display when she was in another area of the store.

Pills and booze hadn't worked for me. But a gun would. I knew Illinois had a law against selling firearms to people with a history of mental illness. And I certainly had a history. But there was also a display on hunting knives nearby. I thought of the scene in *The Godfather II* where a traitor to the family ended his life by cutting his wrists in a warm bath. I could visualize me doing that in our Jacuzzi. I bought one of the knives and hid it once we got home. I told Dr. Francis about the knife and she made me promise to throw it away. I told her I would, but I didn't. The voices telling me to end it all were still very alive inside my head.

Marie decided to do a school health project on manic depression. Dr. Francis agreed to be interviewed by Marie. On the evening of February 13, 1995, Marie asked Dr. Francis questions about bipolar disorder while I videotaped the session.

On February 14, 1995—Valentine's Day—Mark called me from school around noon to tell me he wasn't feeling well. He wanted me to pick him up, but I still didn't have a legal driver's license. I asked him how much money he had. It was enough to take a cab home from school. I told him I would call a cab and that he should wait in front of the school for it. I said I would reimburse him for the taxi fare when he got home.

I jumped out of bed and got dressed. I didn't want my son to know I was still in bed at that time of day.

When Mark got home, he headed straight for the kitchen where he cooked a large frozen pizza in the oven. It looked delicious and I was hoping to have a piece or two, but he ate the whole thing. Normal for a strapping sixteen-year-old boy.

I didn't watch him carefully for the next few hours so I didn't know exactly what he was doing. I know he went to the garage to smoke the cigarettes he wasn't allowed to smoke. And he sat in the family room and read a science fiction book for a while. Then he went back upstairs to his room. Marie had after school activities and came home around 6:30. The phone rang and rang after about a half hour. Marie finally answered it. It was for Mark. She called for him and got no response. She ran up to his room and told him about the call.

I decided to take a shower so I would be somewhat decent when Maura got home from work. The phone rang again. It was Dr. Francis calling to find out if I still had the knife.

If I did she was going to tell Maura about it. Mark answered the phone and told her I was in the shower. They spoke for few moments, and she told him she would call back later.

After my shower the phone rang again. Marie answered it. It was for Mark. Marie called out for him. She ran upstairs and looked through all of the rooms. She couldn't find him anywhere. She ran downstairs and looked all around. Still no Mark. He wasn't on the driveway riding his skateboard.

He wasn't in the garage smoking cigarettes. I heard Marie calling his name over and over and I became alarmed. Even though Mark at times made not being home a science, I became very upset. I felt an overpowering sense of urgency. There were times after school when he practically lived on the phone. It was not like him at all to hide from a phone call. I had to find him.

I ran straight up the stairs to his bedroom. I looked all around and he wasn't there. I walked over to his walk-in closet and tried to open the door. I had to push it hard because I felt a large weight holding the door from being opened. As I pushed as hard as I could, there was a big bump as the door pushed the weight away. With the door finally open, I couldn't believe what I was seeing. Mark was hanging in the middle of his closet, twisting back and forth as a rope was wrapped around his neck and fastened to a high shelf. A river of instant tears rolled down my face. I ran into the closet and put my arms around his waist, holding him up so the rope no longer pulled on his neck. I couldn't leave him. Marie was standing right behind me.

I asked her to run down to the kitchen and bring back a sharp knife. After she brought back a knife, I told her to call 911. "Oh God, please make Mark be alive. Oh Mark, please be alive. Be alive."

We had call waiting and Maura called to say she would be late from work while Marie was on the phone with the 911 operator. "Mark hung himself," Marie told her mother in between deep sobs. "We're afraid he could be dead." When Maura realized Marie was on the line with the emergency operator, she said she would call back a little later.

I cut the rope and gently laid him down on the floor of the large walk-in closet. I knelt over him and tried to administer CPR. I had no training for it. I blew into his mouth and pushed hard on his chest just like I remembered from watching it on television.

Every time I took a breath, I called out for him to still be alive. "Please God, not now, you're too young to die. Please God, not now."

I blew into his mouth as hard as I could, but the air just stayed in his mouth for a moment. It wouldn't go down into his throat. Marie was sitting on Mark's bed still talking to the 911 operator who told her to stay on the line until help arrived. She asked the operator if you could tell Mark was dead because he had wet his pants. We were so scared, so very scared.

As I continued to try to blow air into his lungs, I noticed the shelf he had hung from was not much higher than he had been. When I cut him down, his body seemed to be folded up under him. I thought all he had to do to survive would have been to stand up and relieve the pressure from around his neck.

I hoped he had stood up on his toes to keep the rope from cutting off his air supply. Maybe he hadn't been hanging all that long.

In a few moments the ambulance arrived with police cars and fire trucks. Two paramedics made their way to the closet holding their life saving equipment. "Please step aside, sir, and let us do our job." They asked us to go downstairs and wait. Marie and I sat at our kitchen table holding our breath.

"Mr. Ricke," said a loud voice from Mark's closet. "I'm so sorry. Your son has expired."

I had been the first person to hold him when he came into this world and the last person to hold him when he left.

Marie and I stood up and held onto each other and cried like never before or again.

Maura called back and Marie answered the phone. She could

barely get the words out when she told her mother Mark had died. At first Maura didn't believe it.

She couldn't comprehend the fact her son had killed himself. Because her company's switchboard was closed and we couldn't call her back, the police sent a car to pick her up, but a friend from work drove her home.

As Maura and her friend approached the house, they saw it was surrounded by emergency vehicles. When Maura entered the kitchen she walked toward me past the policemen and firemen who were standing around. Her eyes met mine. They were asking if the nightmare was true, asking me in silence if we had really lost our son. I just nodded my head. Our eyes were still locked as we both wept.

Meanwhile Marie was sitting in an ambulance in the driveway being questioned by police who were concerned that there might be child abuse in the Ricke family.

Our kitchen table was turned into a communications center for the police, paramedics, firemen, and deputies from the county sheriff's office. Every square inch seemed to be covered with portable phones, radios, and battery packs. It gave the impression that those men with their equipment could get you anything in the world that you needed or wanted, anything but your son's life back.

One of the firemen asked us if we would like to talk with the fire department's chaplain. I thanked him for the offer but told him we had our own pastor, Father Jack from St. Anne's Church in Barrington. Father Jack arrived twenty minutes later in a police car with flashing lights and siren. We were totally numb. We just couldn't believe what was happening to our lives.

Father Jack sat with us in the family room and tried to help us. "God didn't kill Mark," he said. "Mark took his own life." I don't remember what else he said. All I could think of was how could the kind and loving God I grew up with allow this to happen?

How? Damn it. How? Nothing Father Jack could say about how bad things happen to good people would answer that basic question. Nothing anyone could say could have lessened the incredible pain and suffering that paralyzed us.

Maura had to see Mark. I had seen him in the closet where I tried to bring him back to life, but Maura had not seen him since she left for work that morning. The police tried to talk her out of it. But she was insistent, and Father Jack told the police to let her see Mark.

The four of us, Maura, Marie, Father Jack, and I, walked up the stairs to see Mark one last time before they took him away. He was inside a black body bag. Someone unzipped it and uncovered him from the waist up.

He was still warm to the touch. Father Jack stood there for moral support. Maura and Marie took turns bathing Mark in tears. I was the last to pay my respects before they took him away. After I knelt by the body bag for a few minutes the police officer gently asked me to move aside. Men from the county morgue were there to take Mark away.

They let me kneel there for a few more minutes before I stood up, and they zipped up the bag and carried him to their truck.

We started to make phone calls. I called my parents who were visiting my sister Kathy in Traverse City, Michigan.

Maura called her sisters in Ireland. We called our family and friends. Later in the evening, I called Dr. Easton and Dr. Francis and left messages with their services.

For the next few days we would tell the story over and over.

Mark hung himself in his bedroom closet. We knew he had been having difficulty at school for a couple of years. We knew he had run away from home to stay with a friend. We knew he had been diagnosed with manic depression. But we didn't know he was anywhere near that depressed or troubled. Not a clue. As far as we knew, he didn't leave a note and he didn't tell anyone that he was thinking of taking his life. The only time suicide came up in his sessions with Dr. Francis was when he told her he hated it for what it had done to his father.

We called and called. People responded immediately. They dropped everything they were doing and got on airplanes or into cars and began their journey to the Ricke home in Barrington, Illinois.

During the next three days while we awaited the results of an autopsy, it seemed like we had to make a hundred decisions. We had to choose a funeral home, the clothes he would be buried in, the coffin, the plot in the cemetery, the liturgical readings for the funeral mass and who would read them, and the flowers. Preparing for the rituals of Mark's death kept us busy. We made lots of phone calls. People started showing up right away. My parents showed up the next morning. The next day Maura's sisters arrived from Ireland.

Early in the morning after Mark died, there was a knock on our front door. We opened it and found Mr. Paggentini, Marie's counselor from middle school, standing there. He was the school official who first suggested Mark see Dr. Francis.

Somehow he had heard the news about Mark's death. He asked for Marie. She was still sleeping. He waited for her so he could comfort her and support her after she woke up.

Friends and family took care of each other while Maura and I did our best to cope with the details of Mark's funeral and burial. My parents and Maura's sisters stayed with us. Most others stayed with neighbors and friends. Some of my family stayed in a local hotel. At the time we didn't know where out-of-town relatives and friends were staying. It was all taken care of. All we knew at the time was that our family and friends were there for us when we really needed them. Some cooked for us and themselves in our kitchen. Neighbors brought us food as they continually asked what else they could do for us.

Dr. Easton put me on a heavier dose of psychotropic medications. We wanted to prevent another hospitalization. I was a zombie, totally numbed from the shock of the suicide and totally medicated to help me deal with it.

We had one night at the funeral home where people could pay their respects. Like everything else at the time, it was a blur. A lot of people came. There was a long line of people waiting to kneel at the side of his coffin. There were scores of young people from

Barrington High School. We had no idea he knew so many students. Our neighbors, relatives and friends were all there close to us.

Dr. Easton came and sat next to me for most of the evening. Dr. Francis came to pay her respects. She was totally shocked by everything including the fact she spoke to Mark only an hour or so before he took his life.

The line of people paying their last respects seemed to stretch out forever in the candlelight of the funeral parlor. There were so many tears on so many faces. No one who knew Mark had any idea he was so troubled. There was no warning. No conversation about wanting to take his life with anyone who knew him. He came home from school early on Valentine's Day and hung himself in his bedroom closet. There was so much grief in that room.

The funeral was at St. Ann's Church the next morning. The ceremonies began at the funeral home where they closed Mark's coffin for the last time. Maura went, but I stayed away because I didn't think I could handle the sight of that lid closing on him forever.

Every night we said bedtime prayers with both of our children. Mark had outgrown it, but Marie still said, "Now I lay me down to sleep, I pray the Lord my soul to keep," every night before she went to bed.

Maura wanted her to recite the prayer at Mark's funeral mass, but Marie just couldn't get a word out. So Maura recited the prayer. She also read some passages of scripture to the audience. Just walking in and nodding my head from time to time was all I could do.

Father Jack gave an eloquent sermon which family members still remember, but I don't. What I remember most was a song called, "On Eagles' Wings." They sang it as the pallbearers carried Mark out of the church into the waiting hearse. The song is about God bringing home loved ones on eagles' wings. I still can cry when I hear that song sung in church.

There was a long line of cars following Mark to the cemetery. I don't know how long, but it seemed to stretch out as far as I could see when I turned my head to watch. At every funeral I remember attending, people always remarked about the long line of cars in the funeral procession as if the length of the line was a measure of the deceased person's popularity. It was no different at Mark's funeral. Everyone was talking about the long line of cars in the funeral procession.

There was another religious service in the cemetery's main building where many of the people in attendance had to stand outside because there was not enough room for them inside. After that ceremony everyone was invited back to St. Ann's church where lunch was served in the basement. Maura, Marie, and I and a handful of others stayed to watch while Mark's coffin was placed in a huge concrete vault and then lowered into the ground. We stood there and watched the men cover the vault with cold February earth. And we knew without saying that our lives would never be the same.

It would take quite some time before the truth of those moments became clear to me.

Yes, Mark was a troubled teen. But his troubles were caused by his mental illness. They were not his fault. He was a just turned sixteen-year-old boy. He lacked any maturity or life experience that could have helped him fight the terrible symptoms of manic depression. I knew how nearly impossible it was for me to keep fighting the terrible suicidal urges manic depression brings its victims. I had been unsuccessful three times in serious attempts to end my life. The closest I got to death was a coma. Mark was successful on his first try.

I'll never know if there was a reason I survived death from manic depression and Mark did not. I would have traded my life for his in a second.

It turns out we did have much in common with our bipolar illness. I was haunted with the delusion that Maura was having an affair. There were times when I was totally consumed by the thought of her with another. I was paranoid. It turns out that Mark thought Carol was seeing some other boy. Was he obsessed like me?

There is a Valentine's Day custom at Barrington High that has boys decorating their girlfriends' lockers. Carol didn't want Mark to decorate her locker. Is that why he came home early? Did that explode the fatal symptom of his bipolar disorder? Did he do it to prove how much she had hurt him? We'll never know, and it really doesn't matter what the trigger might have been, if there even was a trigger. Teenage boys switch girlfriends all the time. Some win time with their sweethearts. Some lose, but no healthy teen takes his life over a high school romance.

Yes, suicide is the second biggest cause of teen death after auto accidents. But I believe that mental illness is a lot more prevalent in teens than we realize, and I believe mental illness breeds most suicides.

There are other tragedies that kill teens. Mark's good friend Kevin died of an accidental drug overdose a few years after Mark lost his life to mental illness.

Chicago Tribune Op-Ed Page
Sunday, June 18, 1995
Celebrating Father's Day Without a Son
By Thomas D. Ricke

Let me tell you about my 13-year-old daughter Marie. I am so proud of her. She gets mostly A's and B's in school. Her fiction entry in the Young Writers Project of the Barrington Arts Council received three 1st place ratings. Marie sings in the Barrington Children's Choir and participates in her school's drama club. She plays a mean game of defense on the soccer field and can run the mile faster than anyone in her class. And she is beautiful.

Marie does all of this just by being herself. She has surrounded herself with good friends who share her values. Marie and I will be spending lots of time together this Father's Day.

On the other hand, this is the first Father's Day that my son Mark and I will not be together. You see my beautiful, strapping,

16-year-old baby boy hanged himself in his bedroom closet on Valentine's Day this year.

I found his body dangling in the closet. While I cut him down, Marie called 911. The pain has been so severe; there's no way to describe it. There was no warning. No note. No one saw it coming, not his counselors and teachers, not his friends, not his family.

Since Mark died, my wife and I have both played the individual recorders in our heads, going over every moment we spent with him since his birth. Were we too strict? Were we too lenient? Should I have quit my job instead of going on all those business trips?

Should I have insisted more often that he go fishing with me? Should there have been more ball games, more hot dogs and hamburgers, more or fewer cigarettes—I don't know; I'll never know. I've played and replayed every conversation I had with him.

When I lost my high-paying job and our family income level went from being in the top 3 percent in America to below the poverty line, should I have tried harder to get another high-powered job? Was he embarrassed with his friends that Dad was staying home and not working?

What did we do wrong? We sent him to the best schools—Immanuel Lutheran, Loyola Academy and Barrington High School. If he were a jar, we tried our best to fill him with good stuff.

Like raising all teens, it wasn't easy with Mark. When he was 14, we discovered he was smoking marijuana on a regular basis so we took him to a hospital in Naperville where there's an excellent substance abuse program for teens.

While he was hospitalized, he was diagnosed with a manic-depressive illness, a medical disorder that's very difficult to spot in teens because the symptoms are not usually severe in teenage years and because normal teenage mood swings and behavior can mask them. Mark spent six weeks in the hospital. When he left he was instructed to keep up two practices to keep stable—take one pill a day and see a therapist once a week.

I am intimately familiar with the symptoms of manic depression. Its gene has been passed in our family. I believed the doctors, but I didn't really see then what I consider now to be manic-depressive behavior in our son.

Night after night he stayed up until 4 a.m. and 5 a.m. watching TV and playing computer games when he had to get up at 6 a.m. for school. Money went through his fingers like water. After a few days he quit the only job he ever had, in the middle of a shift, to go to a concert. He ran away from home. He couldn't sit still for more than a few moments. His friends seemed to plug into his energy either in person or over the phone. At his age, with a phone glued to his ear, his social life meant everything.

He also had more lonely and quiet times. Up in his room, with his music in his ear, he would read two to three books in a row. The day he died he sat quietly in the family room for more than an hour reading science fiction.

Six months before he died Mark decided to stop taking his medication. There was one bad scene in which I tried literally to push it down his throat. But there was no way I could make him take it. At the same time he stopped seeing his therapist. He said he was tired of her "psychobabble." The therapist didn't want us to force him to come.

At the tender ages of 15 and 16 the opinion of your friends means absolutely everything. And during those ages you end up sharing nearly everything about yourself with your friends. Mark did not want to be branded as a "psycho," something he was certain would happen if he continued with his therapy. "Dad," he would say, "you don't know me. I know what I'm doing. I can take care of myself."

In addition to worrying about the stigma attached to his illness, stopping his treatment was a way of saying, "I'm not sick; I don't need help anymore. There's nothing wrong with me." Manic episodes often make people think they're all better.

While every tragedy is different, a friend of mine who is one of Chicago's leading experts in the treatment of manic depression says my son's death was caused by a gene that could have either come from my wife or me, and from my son not taking his medication.

He explained that severe depression in teens can come out of nowhere, with no real explainable reason. Often it lasts for only hours, but no matter how long the young men and women are trapped by it, they see no end. Adults who suffer the same sharp, razor-in-the-brain depression have a sense it can end. Teens don't have that perspective. All they can focus on is making the pain go away.

This Father's Day, I will be thinking of and praying for all of the manic depressive teens who are undiagnosed. The medical profession, the educational establishment, parents and teens, we all need to know the signs of depression and mania in teenagers. We all need to fight the stigma that keeps teens from seeking treatment. This is a completely treatable illness. There's no reason for one teenage suicide, not one.

I'd like to ask a favor of you, the reader. If you're a father or son or daughter, hold each other this Father's Day, hold each other as never before. Think about your whole lives together, where you've been and where you are going.

While I will be spending a lot of time with my daughter Marie, I will have a huge hole in my heart for Mark. On this Father's Day you have each other. And I have a son I will never see again.

———

Mental Health America Bell of Hope Memorial
In Loving Memory of Mark Ricke
February 6, 1979 – February 15, 1995

It's been ten years since I last saw you smile, since I last heard your charming laugh echo through our old hallway. You are sorely missed, Mark, as you always will be. I was too young to realize what was happening within our family, and I am so sorry you were unable to share my veil of ignorance.

When we lost you, I didn't just lose my brother. I lost my protection from monsters in the closet, my secret keeper, my co-host for the radio show we broadcast from your closet, my brave partner in numerous adventures (mainly exploring the unfinished attic) and my best friend. Every grand moment now seems unfinished. Every celebration is bittersweet, marked with the shining glare of your absence.

I don't know how we survived your loss, but life continues and we had to follow suit.

Chapter 10

After Mark died, both Dr. Easton and Dr. Francis insisted I see them every week. Dr. Easton kept me heavily medicated. My doctors, family, and friends all feared that I would self-destruct. In addition to the tremendous grief, I was filled with guilt for bringing suicide into our family only five months before Mark died.

I found myself back in the day program at Rush University Medical Center where a counselor suggested I try volunteering a couple of days a week. She included the National Depressive and Manic Depressive Association (DMDA) located near downtown Chicago in the list of suggested places to volunteer.

I arrived at DMDA offices with a fresh copy of my resume. They immediately accepted me as a volunteer. I started to dress for business and travel to downtown Chicago once or twice a week.

I continued to suffer a series of milder manic episodes that had one thing in common—they caused me to think my wife was having an affair. Maura and I were having problems with intimacy before Mark died. Sex for Maura was nearly impossible after Mark's death. Instead of being understanding about how her tremendous grief could affect her love life, I feared I was losing her to someone else.

When she worked late some nights and I was on the manic side, the fear became fact to me. I was up night after night with the thought of Maura with another man going around and around in my overactive mind like a broken phonograph record.

I began to improve after I started volunteering at DMDA. At first I was slow and somewhat forgetful. But I seemed to get better the longer I volunteered. I was functioning fairly well working two days a week. They had me writing literature for the organization. The op-ed column I wrote for the *Chicago Tribune* about Mark's death didn't take more than a couple of hours to write. The words were right there in my heart. I just had to put them on paper. The words for DMDA came very slowly and painfully at first. I wrote word by word, one at a time. However, I didn't give up, and my writing seemed to improve a little each time I tried it.

About ten months after I wrote the column on Mark's death for the *Chicago Tribune*, DMDA offered me a part-time paying job. I was to be Director of Constituency Services, and I would travel to the office two to three days a week. The job was to manage the national organization's relationship with its more than two hundred chapters all over the US The primary purpose of the job was to answer questions that local chapters may have and to distribute literature they wanted. Although the national organization was run by a small staff and reporting relationships didn't seem to mean much, I would have the help of one very experienced person who reported to me. He worked five days a week so he performed the majority of the work in our area. I continued to function better, but I still had a long way to go before I reached normal.

I had been on Social Security disability for some time because my bipolar illness made it impossible for me to work full time. Now that I was trying to go back to work, I was eligible for what they called the "trial work" program in which I could earn wages and still receive my disability for nine months. If it didn't work out, I would stay the on the disability after the job was lost. The idea was to support efforts to go back to work without penalizing people who tried but were unable to make it back to the workforce.

The co-founder and president of DMD took a liking to me. She tolerated my symptoms, setting an example for other staffers on how to treat me.

Dr. Easton kept changing the combination of my medications trying to make me better. The meds would work some at first but then they would stop working, and I would find myself back in Rush's psychiatric ward. People at DMDA continued to be very supportive of my struggle with manic depression. I continued to improve a little, but I wasn't cured.

A year after Mark's death I became seriously suicidal again. I suffered from a case of dysphoric mania, a combination of mania and depression at the same time.

Mark's death was so very painful to me and my family it is impossible for me to accurately describe the agony. No combination of words could do it, however the horror of Mark's suicide helped keep my death wishes somewhat under control. When I thought of suicide, I could not imagine causing a second dose of suicide's horror for my family and friends. But around the first anniversary of Mark's death, suicide won and I started looking for ways to get a gun. I visited Mark's grave and told him I would soon join him in the afterlife.

Before I was able to find a gun, I called Dr. Easton and he put me back in Rush's psychiatric ward with twenty four-hour one-on-one observation. The years of electric shock treatments started during that hospitalization.

The nurse would wake me about 5:30 a.m. to give me an injection of a tranquilizer. The thought of what was about to happen made me a nervous wreck. Then the loud squeaky wheel of the hospital gurney would wake me again around 6 a.m. They always used the same one. As I heard the wheels get closer and closer, I knew it was coming for me.

The orderly would help me climb onto the cot, and then I would ride lying on my back watching the ceiling lights speed by as the soft, quiet hospital began to wake up all around me. Even with the tranquilizer, I was always extremely nervous about what was going to happen to me when the gurney reached its destination.

I would eventually arrive at a large room where patients were lined up lying on their backs in a long row. ECT at Rush University Medical Center was administered early on Monday, Wednesday, and Friday mornings.

When I was an inpatient I would get three electric shock treatments a week. Over the years I would receive more of them as an outpatient. Then I would arrive at the hospital the night before and leave in the late afternoon on the day I received the treatment. There were times when I would receive the outpatient shock treatments all three days a week. Other times I would get the electric shock treatments once or twice a week.

When I was really doing well I got zapped only twice a month, but that was a rare event in the years I received ECT. Dr. Easton determined how often I would receive the treatments. As much as I hated them, I didn't argue with him.

I trusted him when he told me that we had tried nearly every medicine for manic depression without lasting success and that our last chance to make me better was ECT.

Once I arrived at my station in the large room, an intern or resident would put those sticky round conductors on my chest and stomach and then hook them up to a nearby electric cardiograph machine.

Soon after this, they would put an I.V. into my right arm and hook it up to a bottle of clear fluid hanging from a pole near the front of the cot.

The worst part of the ordeal was lying there waiting for your turn to receive ECT. It felt like I was waiting for my turn to face a firing squad as I heard the loud electric buzzing coming closer and closer as it moved down the line of patients toward me. Waiting for it was much worse than actually getting it.

The goal of the treatment was to create a twenty- to forty-second brain seizure. Just before it was my turn to get zapped, they would inject two medicines into my I.V. line.

One was an anesthetic to make me unconscious so that I would neither feel nor remember the intense ordeal of my brain being jolted by electricity. Before the lights went out, I was always really afraid that I would never wake up after the procedure.

The second drug in the I.V. paralyzed me briefly so that I would not move or even breathe during the treatment. This was to prevent my body from convulsing during the brain seizure. Finally they would put a metal rod on each side of my head and press the switch on the box that sent the electrical current shooting through my brain.

When I awoke in my hospital room a couple of hours later, I would be disorientated and suffer some memory loss. During the outpatient ECTs I would leave the hospital in the late afternoon or early evening and take the commuter train home by myself.

I had to drive myself from the train station to my home. Today they don't let outpatient ECT patients leave the hospital unless they have someone to take them home.

Most patients who receive ECT get a series of a few treatments. I received my first ECT while I was still working at DMDA. My medical caretakers credited the treatments as the main reason for my noticeable improvement. Over the next three years I would receive some 200 electric shock treatments. ECT is becoming more and more popular for patients who don't improve while taking different combinations of psychotropic medications. In my case it's no exaggeration to say they saved my life.

According to much of the literature, ECT can be eighty percent effective, but it can cause short-term memory loss, especially around the time of the treatments. In my case I believe I lost a lot of long-term memory because I received so many shock treatments. I can remember the address of the house where I was raised, but I can't remember much about the years when I received so many electric shock treatments along with heavy doses of several psychotropic medicines.

Dr. Easton kept changing my medicines trying to find the combination that would work best for me. It was not unusual for me to be taking up to six separate medications while I was getting ECT.

But the important fact about the ECT and all the medications at that time was that they made it possible for me to improve both at work and at home. I wouldn't be fully aware of the disabling long-term memory loss until late in 1999 when I had received most of my ECT.

Despite my absences, I was welcome in my new professional home at DMDA. My co-workers knew I had been visiting the hospital for medical treatment quite often, but they didn't know the details of my struggle until I began to speak publicly about my experiences with mental illness.

Meanwhile I continued to get better. I became more dependable. I received ECT as an outpatient for more than a year while I avoided being an impatient locked up in the psychiatric ward on the thirteenth floor at Rush University Medical Center.

As I tried writing speeches for the director and some board members, my skills came back to me. It was like riding a bicycle after a few years of trying in vain to walk or crawl everywhere. "Director of Communications" was added to my title. I was now in charge of the association's literature, including the quarterly newsletter to its national membership, and I was to handle DMDA's relationships with the media.

I had a second person reporting to me. I was still working part-time. I was better than I had been before I went to work at DMDA. I began to feel I was being cured. I went to Weight Watchers and lost fifty pounds. I worked out at the YMCA a couple of times a week. I gave my own speeches to various gatherings of DMDA chapters. I talked openly about my long war with manic depression, and I spoke about my electric shock treatments. I was told that my talks were inspirational to some members. If only Mark could see me now.

As I got better I thought about writing a book like this, but I didn't try to start the project for two reasons. I was afraid of alienating my family and the few friends I had left with the details of my inappropriate behavior. And I didn't remember very much about the worst of times that would come in the last half of 1998 and most of 1999. To write this book I had to spend hours and hours with my caretakers as they would read me notes from our sessions. I read hundreds of pages from hospital records. And I had to interview family members for their descriptions of just how sick I was at various times.

I was ashamed and afraid of getting ECT, but I was grateful that I worked for DMDA. What other employer would allow a staff member to be absent one to three days a week to get electric shock treatments?

DMDA had an impressive record of research about the public's misunderstanding of mental illness, particularly manic depression. Here are some of the survey results I used in preparing speeches, press materials and communications with DMDA chapters:

In 1995 DMDA commissioned a survey by the Rand Corporation of 1,000 randomly selected people that documented just how much bipolar illness is misunderstood.

- Twenty-six percent of the respondents said they
  believed mental illness was caused by childhood
  trauma.
- Twenty-two percent said it was caused by "emotional
  shortcomings."
- Fourteen percent said they didn't know the cause of
  mental illness.
- Only ten percent said they thought mental illness was
  a "physical illness."
- Forty-four percent of young people from age eighteen
  to twenty-four believed that childhood trauma was the
  cause of mental illness, and another twenty-one
  percent of young people said they thought the cause of
  mental illness was "emotional shortcomings." So 65
  percent of the young people surveyed had a total
  misunderstanding of the cause of mental illness.
- Fifty-eight percent of all respondents said they thought
  people could prevent or bring themselves out of the

symptoms of manic depressive illness through self-help techniques. Young people in particular think they can prevent manic depression or somehow snap themselves out of it with positive thinking.

- Thirty-one percent of all respondents believed that manic depression can be self-controlled.
- Twenty-six percent of all respondents said they would feel uncomfortable in the presence of a manic-depressive person.
- Twenty-five percent of those who took the survey believed that manic depressed individuals are personally responsible for the development of their own mood disorders.

DMDA produced two videos that were distributed to its chapters, the media, and anyone who asked for them. Walter Cronkite narrated the first one. The eighteen-minute video about depression was called "Everyone Needs a Hand to Hold On To." The second DMDA video was narrated by Tony Dow. It was called "Dark Glasses and Kaleidoscopes." It was thirty-two minutes long and concentrated on manic depression.

In 1994 DMDA conducted a survey of its members. It found that it took an average of at least eight years of seeking treatment before patients received a correct diagnosis. Patients saw more than three medical professionals before receiving a correct diagnosis. In my case I started to seek professional help in my mid-twenties and did not receive an accurate diagnosis until my mid-forties.

Nearly fifty percent of adults with manic depression were neither employed nor in school. More than fifty percent had financial problems. Nearly sixty percent were going through a divorce or were suffering serious marital difficulties. The survey documented a high percentage of alcohol and drug abuse. And sixty-five percent of patients with manic depression had multiple hospitalizations. As long as I am throwing numbers around, there's the most telling number of all—twenty percent of people with manic depression die from suicide.

My professional life was now wrapped in a worthy cause. I had been involved in causes before. I told true stories as a journalist. I worked on saving New York City from defaulting on its securities. I promoted generous funding of the arts. I managed product publicity and campaigns to improving corporate reputations. But I never had been motivated by such a personal cause. Now I was working to promote public understanding of my mental illness.

The first challenge was to focus on the cause of mental illnesses. Life's horrible moments could certainly trigger an outbreak of mental illness, but life experiences were not the fundamental cause of the disease. I had a wonderful childhood. Although I had asthma for a number of years, I received so much love and support from family and friends I was not permanently affected by the childhood illness. I was able to leave it behind me and get on with my life. Things were really very good until I went away to college and began to self-medicate with alcohol for an illness I wouldn't know I had for another twenty-five years. Mark had a good childhood surrounded by family and friends. He had no real problems until his mental illness kicked in when he was fourteen and killed him days after his sixteenth birthday.

Like cancer or heart disease, mental illness is a physical disease.

Just like a heart can malfunction and flirt with death, the brain can stop functioning normally and flirt with death by suicide. It could be faulty chemistry, a shortage or surplus of the fluids that carry electrical impulses to the billions of cells in a brain. Or the brain could have a physical deformity. I have been told that if you compared my brain scan with the scan of a "normal" person my brain would be noticeably different.

There's heart disease and lung disease and liver disease and all sorts of "diseases." I think it would be more accurate to call mental illness a brain disease. After all, the brain controls a person's thoughts, moods, and behavior. And when the brain is sick or broken one can lose control of mood, thoughts, and behavior. After I began working for mental health non-profit agencies, I discovered that the politically correct term for people with mental illnesses is "consumers."

The idea is that people with a mental illness are "consumers" of mental health medications and therapy. When I think of consumers, I think of people lined up to get in a local Walmart the day after Thanksgiving. I also dislike the term "behavioral health" as a description of what goes on in psychiatric wards.

To me that term implies people with mental illnesses are bad people who choose improper behavior of their own free will. It implies they can control their behavior no matter how sick they are.

Medications can alter a person's brain chemistry and help control the symptoms of mental illness. The right medication or combination of medications can help a patient live a fairly normal life. Extraordinary courage and resolve can make a big difference.

Individual and group therapy can help a lot, but there is no cure for brain diseases, no cure for illnesses such as manic depression or schizophrenia. The only thing you can say for sure about these diseases of the brain is they are totally unpredictable, especially with the fifty percent of people with mental illness who are not getting medical treatment.

There were two main mental health issues at that time. One was to bring more people with mental illnesses into treatment—usually a combination of medication and therapy. Another was what we called "parity." Nearly all health insurance policies had limits on funding medical care for mental illnesses.

Instead of paying eighty or ninety percent of the cost of medical treatment like they do for everything else, many insurance policies paid only fifty percent or less of the cost of medical treatment for mental illnesses. Even Medicare paid only fifty percent of the cost of medical treatment for mental illness while it paid eighty percent for everything else. Then there were annual and lifetime limits on what the policies would pay for the treatment of mental illnesses. While a good percentage of health insurance policies have something like million-dollar lifetime limits on reimbursement for medical care, they had limits of $30,000 or less for mental health care.

They say that medical treatment for mental illnesses improves the lives of eighty percent of those who receive professional care for their brain disease. But only fifty percent or less of people suffering with mental illnesses receive any kind of medical care.

So making affordable high quality medical care for everyone struggling with mental illnesses became another cause.

In the few speeches I gave I spoke about how I was slowly recovering from the symptoms of my manic depression. I talked about the constantly changing combination of medications I was taking and how the latest combinations seemed to be working quite well. I spoke about getting so many electric shock treatments.

I told DMDA members about my frequent battles with suicide and the resulting hospitalizations. I spoke about the huge losses in my life due to bipolar disorder. The loss of my son. The loss of my professional life. I talked about my marital difficulties without going into detail about my failing relationship with Maura.

My story assumed that I was over the worst symptoms of manic depression. With the love and support of my family, with constant electric shock treatments, with group therapy, with individual therapy with both Dr. Francis and Dr. Easton, with medication, and with my own personal determination—with all of this in my favor I believed the worst experiences of my mental illness were behind me. I thought I was really on the mend. I spoke with absolute conviction that this was true.

I also tried to get the audiences to realize that major mental illnesses are quite common. I would read a list of famous people who had suffered from maniac depression, schizophrenia, or unipolar depression.

Some of them are Abraham Lincoln, Virginia Woolf, Lionel Aldridge, Leo Tolstoy, John Keats, Tennessee Williams, Vincent Van Gogh, Isaac Newton, Eugene O'Neill, Charles Dickens, Ernest Hemingway, Sylvia Plath, Michelangelo, Jimmy Piersall, Patty Duke, Winston Churchill, Beethoven, Vivien Leigh, Walter Cronkite, and Ted Turner, just to name some of the famous people who were able to make huge contribution to society despite or because of their mental illness.

My sense of near-total recovery at that time was wishful thinking on my part, but there was no doubt that I was getting better. After all, I was working an average of three days a week and doing quite well. I still went to the Y on a regular basis. I attended Weight Watchers. I continued to take part in group therapy programs. I still saw Dr. Easton and Dr. Francis frequently. And I never missed a dose of the many medications I was supposed to take.

Even though I was functioning better, I exhibited symptoms of my illness that Dr. Easton and Dr. Francis noticed. But they were not as serious as they had been before Mark's death. I tried my best to stay focused on the positive elements of my life at that time. I told everyone who would listen to me that I was nearly cured from mental illness. I still cried sometimes when no one else was around to see me, but I tried to keep those waves of utter sadness over Mark's suicide to myself. I wanted everyone to think the worst symptoms of my brain disease were over for good.

As much as I wanted Maura to think that I was practically cured she didn't buy the story I was telling everyone who would listen to me. She experienced Tom Ricke after work and saw that I still struggled with some symptoms of my manic depression. She worried about how Mark's death would affect what she saw as my ongoing "fragile state."

Meanwhile Marie did her best to try and cope with her grief over losing her brother to suicide. She feared she would never be happy again. She worried that Maura and I would divorce. She was very concerned about what other children thought about her in the wake of her brother's tragic death. Most of all, she felt guilty that she survived her brother.

Looking back, Maura and I were so consumed with our grief we didn't pay enough attention to our daughter and how she was struggling to overcome her terrible pain over Mark's suicide and her fear of what would happen to her if her parents divorced.

Marie tried her best to stay focused on school and her friends. She gave her presentation on bipolar illness focusing on the video we recorded with Dr. Francis the night before Mark died. She continued her singing in the Barrington Choir where she sang like an angel as one of the group's featured voices. The choir had an excellent, well-earned reputation. It performed in London and at Carnegie Hall in New York City. She had important roles in the high school's plays. She ran as fast as anyone in her class, and she earned mostly all A's. She started to date about the time she turned sixteen. Despite her great grades, substantial extracurricular activities, and close friends, Marie wished she had a punching bag in her room. Her anger would have her destroying it.

While I was working at DMDA, Maura and I attended meetings of a group called "LOSS," which stood for loving outreach for survivors of suicide. It was a pretty big group of family members who were suffering from the suicide of a loved one. The program was run by a Catholic priest but was open to anyone suffering from another's self-willed death. Maura and I found it helpful to talk to people going through the same pain and sorrow that we were experiencing. I was surprised to see so many people from every walk of life had experienced the suicide of a loved one.

I was also surprised to learn that a very large percentage of the suicide victims suffered from mental illnesses. The largest group of suicide victims suffered with bipolar disorder, but there also were victims with schizophrenia and unipolar depression. I can't remember a single suicide not caused by a mental illness. The strongest human instinct is to live, to hang onto our lives with every bit of our mind and body. When a person's thoughts, words, and actions are overcome by suicidal impulses, those impulses can become stronger than the will to live. This is pure insanity. There's no other way to accurately describe suicide. It's insanity. As they say, it's a "permanent solution to a temporary problem."

I continued to perform in the office. I developed relationships with my co-workers and people who ran local chapters of DMDA. The pharmaceutical industry makes a lot of profit on medicine for psychiatric conditions. And the drug companies generously offer financial support to non-profit mental health agencies. Some of the support is for specific programs, and some of it is for general purposes.

I developed relationships with the representatives of some of those companies. My closest relationship was with the manager of public affairs at Eli Lilly.

One day our executive director just disappeared. The gossip said she had a severe attack of manic depression, and she just left her home and her office. No one who worked on the DMDA staff knew what happened to her. No one knew how to reach her. If anyone knew the truth it would have been the leadership of the board of directors, but if they knew, they weren't telling anyone.

After several months of her absence the board started a formal process to choose another executive director. I decided to throw my hat in the ring.

My experience made me an expert on manic depression. I had an inspiring story to tell. I didn't think it hurt that I had good management and public relations experience.

I began to collect letters of support from people I used to work for and doctors in the mental health field, including Dr. Easton and Dr. Francis. I went on a personal campaign to convince everyone that I could be a fine executive director of DMDA. I asked them to believe that my personal determination and my willingness to do whatever my caretakers asked me to do had put me on the road to a remarkable recovery.

I must have been very convincing because I received support from bosses and co-workers from everyplace I worked since my first suicide attempt.

Former CEO of Philip Morris Companies, Inc., Hamish Maxwell, wrote an extremely positive letter about my experience and ability. I also had an impressive list of people who agreed to be a reference for me. The list includes Kay Redfield Jamison, author of *An Unquiet Mind,* a very popular book about her own struggles with manic depression and suicide. She is a doctor of psychology and a professor at Johns Hopkins School of Medicine. She has written several other books about mental illness and suicide including co-authoring the textbook on manic depression used in medical schools. It would take another chapter to accurately describe her work and all the national awards she has received for it.

Stanley Brezenoff, former President of the New York City Health and Hospitals Corporation, was also on my list of references, as was Bob Laird from the editorial board of the *New York Daily News*.

The two top executives on the DMDA staff at the time, acting Executive Director Donna DePaul-Kelly and Director of Administrative Services Rose Armstrong agreed to serve as references for my candidacy.

I felt somewhat confident about my chances of getting the job. I believed my own hype that I had unique media and political experience as well as high-level corporate experience that other candidates would be hard pressed to match. All of my suffering with manic depression including the loss of Mark could be used to help others with mental illnesses.

On the other hand I had no experience in raising funds for a non-profit agency, and the only managing experience I had in the non-profit arena was my rather recent and limited experience at DMDA. I was still receiving electric shock treatments, and I wasn't working full-time.

I wrote a three-page letter to members of the board of directors. It basically said that my employment history and my personal history with manic depression made me a terrific candidate for the executive director position. I also outlined my vision for the future of DMDA including expanding its corporate funding base beyond the pharmaceutical industry's support and offering better programs of support to its chapters. I don't remember much about my interview with the board's search committee other than the sense that I had performed quite well.

We heard from the board a few months after my interview. They chose a woman with a history of very good administration experience to be DMDA's next executive director. My colleagues at DMDA were supportive of me after the choice was announced. I was disappointed, but I still had an important job at the association. I could be a big help to my new boss.

After a few months she called me into her office and fired me. I believe the DMDA board passed me over because I had manic depression, and its members feared what could happen to the organization if I became extremely ill. DMDA's founder disappeared after a serious episode with her illness. What would Tom Ricke do if his illness acted up? They all knew my story, so they knew how sick I had become in the past. I know it sounds somewhat strange that a national organization devoted to supporting people with depression and manic depression would pass over a qualified candidate because he had manic depression. But I believe that's exactly what happened. Knowing what I do today about my mental illness at that time, I would have made the same decision about me.

I didn't pay too much attention to DMDA after I left. The new executive director must have performed pretty well. The organization continued to be a big help to its chapters. It continued its national conferences on important mental health issues. One action I did notice what that it changed its name from the National Depressive and Manic Depression Association (DMDA) to the more politically correct Depression and Bipolar Support Alliance (DBSA).

Chapter 11

A fter I lost my job at DMDA, I feared my life would be an endless series of empty days.

With Marie in school and Maura at work, I was alone in our house for most of the day.

With nothing to do I could sleep until any hour, and during that time I often slept until noon or later. And, of course, there were times when I didn't sleep at all.

A public relations agency in New York City began giving me freelance work. I would wait until the last minute to finish a project, but I did the work, and they accepted it and paid me for it. I set up an office in a room on the first floor of our house. We had moved to a smaller house near downtown Barrington because living in the house where Mark died was just too painful for us.

Even though I had been getting better, I was still basing my self-esteem more on my unhappy relationship with Maura than anything else.

There was absolutely no affection. I thought she was crabby and cranky and critical of me. Now I think I understand what was happening then. Before Mark died she was turned off by some of the nasty symptoms of my illness. After Mark died, my long, severe history of suicidal thinking and behavior scared the love and affection right out of her. Mark's death tortured her with indescribable pain and suffering. Making love to me would be terribly dangerous. It would make her feel so close to me that if I were to die from suicide, she would never be able to recover.

To stay safe from that unimaginable level of pain she had to stay away from me any way she could.

Of course, it would have been impossible for Maura to shield herself from the emotional consequences of my suicide no matter how she treated me. At that time we had been married for twenty-two years, and her instinct for self-preservation must have been stronger than any feelings of love she still may have had for me.

From time to time she would blame me some for Mark's suicide. Not only did I bring suicide into the house the year before Mark died, I should have found him in his closet sooner.

She also thought she spent too much time looking after me and not enough time with Mark. If only she had spent more of her time and attention with Mark, she may have been able to save him.

Now and again she would think of divorce, but the Irish in her resisted it.

Despite the electric shock treatments I still received and the noticeable loss of balance that was a side effect of my medications, I rode my big Honda all over the place. Occasionally I would lose my balance and drop the motorcycle when I was stopped.

I drove it to Detroit to visit my brother and parents. I took I-94 all the way. Mr. Easy Rider. Mr. Sex Appeal. Wind in my face and the hot powerful engine between my legs. If my sexual relationship with Maura had been normal, would I have purchased the big machine? Probably not. Even though I had good reason to fear falling down or falling off, I still rode it. It was a challenge to my manhood.

I drove all the way back to Chicago. When I pulled into the crowded Michigan rest stops to relieve myself, I tried to notice how the nearby women were looking at me.

Could I be their Clint Eastwood? Their Marlboro Man?

A few weeks after the trip, I received a phone call from the executive director of the Mental Health Association in Illinois (MHAI). The manager of community relations for Eli Lilly gave the association a $25,000 grant so she could hire me part-time.

This happened because of the good relationship I developed with Eli Lilly when I worked at DMDA. So my work at DMDA wasn't all in vain. It ended up really helping me when I needed something good to happen in my part-time professional life.

I started a couple of weeks later. I liked the people there, but in the beginning there wasn't much for me to do. I started planning and writing the Association's newsletter. I was receiving Social Security disability again, and I couldn't earn more than $500 a month or I would lose the disability benefits which included Medicare. Despite my somewhat successful stint working part-time at DMDA, both Dr. Easton and Dr. Francis warned me that I should not work full-time at MHAI. I never worked a forty-hour week at DMDA. I was still taking several different medications, and I was still receiving electric shock treatments. They believed the pressures of working full-time would almost certainly put me back in the psychiatric ward of Rush University Medical Center.

Maura, Marie and I spent three weeks in Ireland over the Christmas holidays that year. I thought it was a great trip. I fantasized that our troubles were going to be over when we got home. I had a new, secure job at MHAI.

My fantasy about a better relationship with Maura disappeared soon after we got home. My self-confidence took another nose-dive. She always seemed to be angry with me.

It wasn't her fault, but I found myself slipping into a nasty depression. Everything was dark and difficult. Just about anything hurt me deeply.

I was lying face up on the gurney again as the male nurse pushed me down to the big room where they administered ECT. It was just like all of the other times. They put the I.V. in my arm and I waited for them to administer the anesthesia. After they did, I was unconscious while they added the medicine that would paralyze me for a few minutes.

They were just about to give my brain the electrical shock

when I woke up. They didn't give me the right dose of anesthesia. I couldn't move. I couldn't breathe. I fought the paralysis with all my strength and determination. I began to flop on the table like a fish out of water. I tried to scream, but nothing came out. It was a wide-awake nightmare. No matter how hard I tried, I couldn't breathe. I felt as if I were suffocating. I felt like I was dying right on that table. They gave me another dose of anesthesia and I was soon unconscious again for the rest of the procedure. When I awoke in my hospital room a couple of hours later, there was a nurse sitting near the bottom of my bed. She took my vitals which must have been okay because she left the room.

I found myself back at Rush a few weeks later, but this time I was on a medical floor. I had a terrible pain in my lower left leg caused by rather large blood clots. If they got loose and ended up in my lungs or heart or brain, all my depressive dreams of leaving this earth could have come true.

They tell me I wasn't scared, but I remember lying there fantasizing what it would be like for a clot to get loose. Would a clot to the lungs make it impossible to breathe like the ECT-gone-bad incident? What would a heart attack feel like if a clot reached mine? And if it made it to my brain would the resultant stroke cripple me for life or kill me?

I knew I was in an excellent hospital with a very good doctor overseeing my treatment.

There was nothing else I could do to save my life. They told me I would have to be on Coumadin forever. I still take it today, and the bottom third of my left leg is still all deep purple with red blotches that keep me from wearing shorts. No more clots, but permanent skin damage from when they were there.

Not too long after I came home from the hospital, I started going to the strip clubs again. This time I put a thousand-dollar roll of bills in my pocket and made sure the young women could see it. I wasn't trying to get laid. I was probably impotent at the time. I would discover later that the embarrassing and frustrating inability to have sex was a side effect of the medication I was taking and probably would have to take for the rest of my life. Dr.

Easton gave me samples of Viagra. I was lucky. I wouldn't have the opportunity to use it for at least a year, but when I did it worked its magic, and I functioned normally—whatever that is.

Apparently I was just looking for female companionship in these bars where well-heeled patrons paid a good amount of money to have a young woman dance privately for them. Apparently I was willing to give big tips for the private entertainment.

The thousand-dollar roll of hundred-dollar bills got thinner and thinner. Dr. Francis thought I was manic and threatened to tell Maura if I continued to waste money on strippers.

One young woman met me for lunch outside of the club where she worked. She told me about her young child at home and how his father took off just before he was born.

I told her all about my life with Maura and described my mental illness. She seemed genuinely interested. I left the lunch on my motorcycle hoping that image would make her more interested in me, but she moved to another club and I never saw her again.

Dr. Francis's notes from a session around that time said that although I was manic and obsessing over the stripper I really wanted to be closer with Maura.

In June of 1998 I had my last motorcycle ride. I don't remember the accident. The police thought that I must have been run off the road into a ditch by a driver who kept going. I've often wondered if I lost control of the machine all by myself.

They had to cut the helmet from my head. My motorcycle was in pieces scattered over the ground near Route 22 where I was riding. I was in a coma again. This time it lasted for several days.

When I awoke, I found out that I had suffered a serious concussion. I had bleeding inside of my brain. Nearly all of my right-side ribs were broken. A brain scan showed I had brain damage that could be permanent. My balance had been poor before the accident. Now it was really bad. I had to walk with a cane for several months.

About a month after my hospitalizations for the motorcycle accident I found myself back on the thirteenth floor of the Rush University Medical Center again receiving three shock treatments a week for two weeks. Dr. Easton was trying to knock a nasty depression out of my damaged brain.

Here are some quotes from my 1998 hospitalization reports:

He has suicidal ideation and he could not sleep for the past two nights. The patient was shaking in the bed. The whole day he was crying for no apparent reason. . .

He says his life is worthless. He has no energy for work. He has poor concentration. His appetite is decreased. He was having anhedonia and suicidal ideations. . .

The patient's speech was soft, slow and monotonous, very poor eye contact, motor, psychomotor. The patient had a fine tremor in both hands. His mood was very, very depressed.

His speech was somewhat rapid. All movements were slow and halting. Eye contact was sporadic. His motor functions were very slow with an ataxic quality.

Very poor fine motor control when writing, also very unsteady when walking. His affect was constricted and his mood was described as anxious and irritable. His speech showed increased rate. His thinking was disorganized.

He was frequently distracted and derailed. He had paranoid delusions about his wife trying to steal his money.

The patient had a very unsteady gait. The patient was shuffling, falling to both sides.

The patient is also with positive Romberg and unable to do heel to toe walking.

The patient on admission was confused, disoriented and his memory and concentration were poor. His motor functions were slow with an abnormal gait and possible right facial droop. His speech was slow and his mood was blue.

The patient complains of sleep disturbances and feelings of helplessness and hopelessness. He doesn't feel he has anything to look forward to.

So during the first eight months of 1998 I had been hospitalized for dangerous blood clots, a concussion with noticeable brain damage, and my ongoing mental illness.

I moved in slow motion, and I would continue to do so for years to come. My reaction to everything was very slow. This affected my driving. After scaring them with close calls, Maura and Marie wouldn't let me drive when they were in the car. Marie was in her senior year in high school and didn't want me going with her and Maura to look at colleges.

I went back and forth about Maura. I would try to be supportive of her realizing she too suffered from depression after Mark died. I would tell myself that she stood by me in the beginning of my mental health issues. The least I could do was to support her and be understanding about her lack of interest in intimacy with me. I tried, but before long I would be convinced she was being intimate with someone else.

Today I know she was faithful to me during that time, but then I was tortured with the frequent delusion that she wasn't.

I would have another medical emergency before the year was over.

The side effects of my medicine caused me to lose my balance and take a bad fall in our bathroom. I broke some of my ribs again.

They took x-rays and found a mass on my ribs that was consistent with cancer. A few days later they did a bone scan. I went to work the next day where I had a hard time concentrating on anything. I was more worried and upset over this finding than I was with my blood clots or my suicidal times. Years before when we lived in New York I had another cancer scare. I had a big bump on the back of my head that was a bone tumor. It turned out to be non-malignant, but they took it out anyway because it could have changed.

Finally, they did a biopsy on the growth on my ribs and determined the mass was a non-malignant result of the motorcycle accident. After the good news, Maura and I spent a weekend in downtown Chicago. Then she went to Ireland for a couple of weeks with a plane ticket I gave her for her birthday.

On December 7 I showed up for a session with Dr. Francis in a severe depression. I told her I had no purpose in life. I wanted to hang myself to experience what Mark did. I told her I would do it after I got home. She determined that I was serious and could not guarantee my safety after I left her office. She called Dr. Easton. He arranged a bed for me in my second home.

Dr. Francis called Maura, and they agreed that I couldn't be trusted to drive downtown to Rush. I would leave the car in Francis's parking lot and take a taxi to the Rush emergency room where they would be waiting for me. After it arrived, Dr. Francis walked with me to the taxi to be sure I got in it. It was at least an hour drive from Francis's office to Rush.

In those years there were times when I practically lived in the psychiatric wards of Rush University Medical Center. There were four separate wards. I spent most of my time in the large, locked ward on the thirteenth floor where two to three patients shared each room. There were two television rooms and a large day room where meals were served and patients met with visitors. When Maura visited me she would take my arm and walk around and around the circle shaped ward.

There were two psychiatric units on the twelfth floor. One was for the very ill patients who required more attention and security than the patients on thirteen. When I was very ill I would stay in that ward.

What I remember most about my visits was standing in line to get a light for my cigarettes. There was a hole in the wall where a hot element of some sort lit the patients' smokes. They let you have a cigarette every half hour. So there was a nearly constant line for the hot hole in the wall. I remember looking at other patients on that unit and thinking these people are really, really sick. It didn't occur to me that I was just like them. There were times in 1998 and 1999 that doctor Easton told me I was "as sick as you could get" from my mental illness.

On the other half of the twelfth floor there was a unit that was not locked and mostly used for detoxing alcoholics. I would stay there on the nights before my outpatient electric shock treatments when I was not ill enough for the locked wards.

I would leave in the late afternoon after my ECT. They called it a twenty three-hour admission. I took the train from Barrington to downtown Chicago and back all by myself.

Two weeks and six shock treatments later I was released. The shock treatments did their job. After I got home, I told Dr. Francis I was extremely grateful to her for saving my life.

The executive director of MHAI was very understanding during those times of frequent hospitalizations. She kept my job waiting for me no matter how much time I missed for medical emergencies.

If you count the times I stayed overnight for outpatient shock treatments in 1998, I had at least twenty hospitalizations plus the cancer scare. I would receive a total of some 200 electric shock treatments before they were stopped in 2001.

At the end of all my hospitalizations in 1998 I was looking forward to 1999. I figured it would have to be much better than the year before. But I was wrong.

Chapter 12

I spent most of December 1998 in Rush's psychiatric wards. I came home for the holidays, but I wasn't there for very long. They told me my illness had become "organic." My reactions were so very slow. I drifted from side to side as I shuffled along in slow motion. I couldn't remember anything. I had severe motor issues, and suicide called to me day and night. As Maura tried to build a stronger wall of emotional distance between us the urge to die became more intense.

I was as depressed as I had ever been. We had so many happy holidays when the four of us were a family together. But this Christmas was as cold as the snow and ice outside.

On January 4, 1999, I tried a new way to end my life. My attempt with taking lots of liquor and pills put me into comas, but they didn't kill me. They were failures. Each time I was angry to be alive when I gained consciousness. I didn't want to make that same mistake again. It would take a truckload of pills to end my life. So I tried carbon monoxide instead. Ending the horrific pain that made every thought and movement unbearable became more urgent than my concerns about how much pain my suicide would cause my family and friends.

I sat in my car with the motor running, the windows open and the garage door closed. Again, I wanted to fall asleep and never wake up.

After ten or fifteen minutes Marie opened the door to the kitchen and ran out to my car. "Daddy, what are you doing? Stop it. Stop it now," she screamed.

I told her to mind her own business and to leave me alone. She ran back into the house to find Maura. The woman who was legally still my wife marched into the garage coughing with her hand over her mouth. She raised the garage door.

Then she walked over to the car, opened the passenger door, sat down and yanked the keys from the ignition. Why wouldn't they just let me die?

Soon I was back in the psychiatric ward at Rush. I was under a twenty four-hour watch. At night they dragged my bed next to the nursing station where they could watch me every minute.

Just after the garage attempt, Maura promised herself she wouldn't delay the divorce any longer. There was a tragic story in the news then. A man killed himself the same way I tried to. He was successful and died in his car. The engine kept running for a long time and carbon monoxide crept under the door to the house eventually killing his wife and two children as well. Maura was very afraid that the same thing could happen to her and Marie.

I was in Rush for a long time after the carbon monoxide attempt. My parents came to visit me. Maura was still extremely upset about my attempt in the garage so my father installed a carbon monoxide alarm over the kitchen door which led to the garage.

When my parents came to visit me at Rush I didn't recognize them at first. However, once I remembered who they were, their love and support made me feel better.

I lived on the twelfth and thirteenth floor at Rush much of the time between December of 1998 and April of 1999. Dr. Francis's notes from our session on January 27 said, "Organic slow reactions, memory lapses, motor problems so bad."

On February 2 she wrote: "Looks like a zombie so heavily medicated can't drive, sleeps all day, doesn't remember suicide attempt in hospital when he tried to hang himself with his belt like Mark. Gone for two months in Rush."

During the first week in April after I came home from the long stay at Rush, I immediately felt almost happy dreaming that our love life was back on track. I missed the obvious signs that the marriage was close to being over.

Maura was very frustrated that I only talked about sex when our lives were "in shambles" and I hadn't acknowledged what she's been through for the past ten years. I would tell her the only thing worse than living with mental illness was having mental illness.

In the autumn of 1999 the three of us attended my niece Sarah's wedding in Detroit. Marie was in the wedding ceremony. All my brother and sisters were there with their families.

Maura used the occasion to tell everyone in my family that she had made up her mind to divorce me. So I found out about her plan to file for divorce second-hand. She had threatened to leave me before, but this was the first time she said she was going the end the marriage. It wasn't a threat. It was a fact. She had the name and number of an attorney, and she planned to set up an appointment with him. I was totally devastated. I sat by myself in a corner until my sister Peggy came over to comfort me. I sat with her for the remainder of the event. The ride home to Chicago with Maura and Marie was horrible. I felt very bad about Marie. She was caught in the middle of it all.

It would take me a lot longer to accept the reality of the impending divorce. Maura didn't file right away so I told myself that she was changing her mind. I changed the focus of my fear from the absence of intimacy to living alone with no one to care for me when the madness took over.

For several years our family had been having reunions each July. In 1999, we celebrated my parents' fiftieth wedding anniversary by renting cottages around a lake in Canada near to where my sister Sue lived with her family. I had just returned to the real world after another stay at Rush. I still walked off balance shuffling my feet from side to side. I was 6'2" and looked my best at around

210 pounds. That summer I weighed 168 pounds. I was really skinny and very shy.

At that time I had significant difficulty interacting with others —even my own family.

I got totally confused at O'Hare airport where I was to board a plane to Toronto. I waited for quite a while in the long line for domestic flights until I realized there was another long line for international flights not far away. I walked over to the end of the international line. It wasn't very long before I began to panic. I didn't know where I was supposed to be. How do I get to the gate? I was afraid I was still in the wrong place and would end up missing my flight.

I saw a woman wearing an airline uniform walking nearby. I left my space in line and ran over to her. I told her I was mentally ill and very confused about what to do to catch my flight. She must have realized I was telling her the truth. She walked me to the front of the line and then took me to the gate where I would board the plane.

My sisters and brother each stayed in cottages with their families. Since I was there by myself, my parents rented a two-bedroom cottage so I could stay with them. In the evenings my siblings sat around a campfire drinking a few beers and remembering their young lives in Detroit. A couple of my older nephews joined them.

I stood by the window in my bedroom in my parents' cottage where I could hear them talking. I was too shy and sensitive to join them. I knew they loved me. They didn't mean to treat me differently, but they did. I was the mentally ill member of the family. I was really bad with multiple hospitalizations and more than 150 electric shock treatments at that time.

I was so crazy I was receiving Social Security disability. I walked like an old man with impaired balance. When I did speak, I talked so softly it was hard to hear what I was saying. Instead of taking a chance they would upset me and cause me to somehow relapse they didn't say much to me, and when they did they spoke to me as if I were a child.

I felt like a child. My siblings were there with their children. I was by myself staying with my mom and dad just like when I was a child suffering with asthma.

I remember joining my family for two activities.

We went horseback riding. I got a very gentle horse but my balance was not good and I had great difficulty staying in my saddle. When they got their horses to go faster I stayed behind struggling to stay on my horse as it walked slowly. I couldn't wait to get off the horse and go back to my room.

A few of us went to play golf. I figured that with all the golf I had played I would not embarrass myself. But I did and picked up my ball after a few holes. I was slowing everyone down looking for my ball which never landed near the fairway.

After I returned home I resumed my part-time job at MHAI, but it was not easy at first. I remember standing in front of the Xerox machine wondering where to put the paper when a co-worker had to show me how it worked.

I was making "over-the-phone friends" with the staff of the National Mental Health Association (NMHA) in Washington, DC. The national headquarters for our organization was really improving. It had been near bankruptcy for several years. Under new management it was receiving lots of contributions and it regained much of its political influence involving national mental health issues. I met the new president when he visited our office in Chicago. We seemed to like each other. Because it was doing so well financially NMHA was hiring new people. There was one open job for someone to manage media relations. I was told that if I applied for it I would have an excellent chance of being hired. I told Maura about it.

She told me she hoped that I would get the job because it would give me a chance to start over. I finally got the nerve to ask the question I was afraid to ask. "Would you come with me?"

"No," she answered.

I knew she was planning to divorce me, but I had hoped the new opportunity would make her think twice about the divorce.

The "no" hit me like a bullet in the heart. I never did get the opportunity to interview for that job. Once they discovered I was still receiving electric shock treatments they lost interest in me.

I had been asking Maura for years to join me in a session with Dr. Francis. I thought it would be like marriage counseling. I thought it could save our marriage if it went well. When Maura finally agreed to join me and Dr. Francis I was so happy. I really thought that if anyone could save our marriage it would be Ruth Francis. About halfway through the session Dr. Francis asked Maura a general question about our marriage. I will never forget Maura's answer: "I don't love him the way he wants me to." It was the final death knell for our marriage. The session I wanted gave Maura the opportunity to tell me she didn't love me anymore in the safety of Dr. Francis's office. Even though we were still living together, it wasn't long before Maura started a campaign to convince me to date others. I suppose she would have less guilt if I was with someone else. I tried to meet someone online. It wasn't working so I ended up signing with a dating service for $1,100.

I told Maura about it, and she called the service, told them I was mentally ill, and got them to cancel the fee on my credit card. Her pushing me to date someone else was killing me, but I wanted to please her, and I didn't want to end up all alone so I kept trying.

The first singles event I attended was an evening of bowling. There were at least twice as many women there than men. I met Evelyn, a pretty blonde real estate agent. I was shy, but she still gave me her card and told me to call her. On our first date Evelyn wanted to pick me up at my house. I told her Maura had filed for divorce and I was going to leave her soon.

She parked her car on the street in front of our house. I walked out and got into her car. Before we left Maura ran out of the house toward the car. "He is a good person," she yelled, "He is a good person."

"What's that all about?" Evelyn asked as we pulled away. I didn't know what to say. We went out a few times and eventually became lovers. I was so surprised because I had told her about my illness and she still wanted to be with me. She took a Saturday off to help me find an apartment so I would have a place to stay when

Maura and I finally split up. She brought me to a large apartment complex located not too far from where I was living. It wasn't the nicest place we looked at, but it was near where I already lived, and I was familiar with the area. Just after Evelyn found the apartment for me she told me she couldn't see me anymore because she and her former boyfriend were getting back together. I was disappointed but not devastated. We certainly weren't in love, and I had already met someone else before Evelyn and I split up.

There was a restaurant called the Barn of Barrington. It held dances for singles on Friday and Saturday nights. I met Jane there. Jane was a music teacher and widow who was missing the affection and attention of a good relationship. We got along well from our very first dance.

She tolerated me talking about my problems with Maura, and my history of mental illness didn't scare her away. I would even bring my nighttime medicines with me when we were in her house so I wouldn't forget to take them.

After I left the house Maura and I shared, Jane and I went to several concerts of the Chicago Symphony Orchestra at Ravinia, the outdoor concert venue, where we would sit on a blanket and have an evening picnic while we listened to the music.

We saw each other at least once a week. I often brought her flowers. I wanted to sleep all night with her, but it just wasn't going to happen. She didn't feel comfortable on the waterbed in my apartment, and she didn't want her neighbors to see a male friend's car in her driveway all night. She was a music teacher, and she was afraid that tarnishing her reputation would hurt her business.

I didn't mind. I was grateful for her company. Seeing her helped my state of mind in dealing with the difficult divorce with Maura. In fact, seeing Jane helped my self-esteem during those painful days. I don't know how I would have made if without her affection and understanding. I especially liked it when she played the violin for me.

Maura wanted total control of a fund to pay for Marie's out-of-state college room, board, and tuition. I wanted to pay for all of

Marie's college, but Maura was asking for at least $30,000 to $40,000 more than it would actually cost.

I didn't like not having any input in how the funds were spent. We compromised. We set a lower amount aside but agreed that we would increase it equally should the actual costs be more. Maura would have control of the fund, but she would inform me how it was being spent. I'm sure my ongoing mental illness was a big factor in keeping me away from Marie's college funds. In the years to come, Maura did not let me know the details of the fund's expenditures. I didn't like it, but I decided not to make a big issue of it. There was no way that Maura would misuse the funds set aside for Marie's higher education.

What really upset me was splitting up my pensions. I had enough pension funds from both Philip Morris and Kraft to retire comfortably.

But according to Illinois state law a woman who stays at home caring for her family gets half of her husband's pension. I understand the reason for the law, but I just didn't like what it did to me.

Moving day finally arrived. We were still arguing about terms of the divorce, but we both knew it was time to actually live apart. Maura had already decided what I would take with me. I had boxed up all of my writing that I still possessed. I took two items that had been in my family for generations. One was a hand-carved pre-Civil War loveseat. The other was a big oak table with chairs like thrones that came from my father's parents. It was about a hundred years old. Maura wept while the movers were putting my things on their truck.

She wanted to have dinner with me that night, but Dr. Francis told me not to go with her. I had dinner with Jane instead.

It was dark and quiet and lonely in my new apartment. I had a hard time falling asleep in the beginning. I would watch television until I couldn't keep my eyes open and then crawl into the waterbed. On the nights I couldn't sleep I would read as long as I could and watch rented movies. I often felt alone living with Maura, but not this alone.

I was quoted in an article in the Chicago Tribune. It identified me as a spokesperson for MHAI. On the day the article appeared I got a phone call from a woman who remembered me from Rush. Julie told me we had been patients at Rush together. We talked for a while and agreed to have lunch the next day.

She was a pretty, thin blonde who made me feel comfortable right away. She told me that when we were patients at Rush, she wished she could be Maura. Julie saw Maura walking me around and around in the ward.

Julie told me she knew that Maura and I had children and lived in the suburbs. Julie lived in the city by herself. She said she wanted to be my wife, but that was some sort of delusion. She had a terrific smile. We went to the Art Institute together and we had lunch a few more times. She gave me one of my favorite quotes: "I may be crazy, but I'm not stupid." I used that quote in Maura's attorney's office when I was handed a check for my portion of the proceeds from the sale of our house that was short of what is should have been.

I must have spent a lot of time with Julie complaining about how badly Maura treated me. I must have talked about how I couldn't believe Maura dumped me. I must have told her how unhappy I felt. Her second memorable quote was "I'm not Mother Theresa." That's what she said when she told me she didn't want to see me anymore.

I regret bitching so much about my life. Julie and I had a lot in common. We were both patients of Dr. Easton. We both were attractive and intelligent. We liked each other, but the odds were against us. It is probably very difficult for two mentally ill people to have a romantic relationship. Yes, they most likely could both understand each other's craziness, but that doesn't mean they could live with it.

When one—or even both—of them had strong mental symptoms, their relationship would be nearly impossible to survive. Still, I would have liked to have given it a better chance than we did.

Jane and I had dinner together the night before I had to be in court to make the divorce with Maura official. It was awful. She used the occasion to let me know that she wanted us to be "just friends." No more sex and affection.

It was a knock-out punch. I suspect the fact that I was experiencing symptoms and still getting electric shock treatments might have scared her away. I lost Jane that night, and I was going to officially lose Maura in a divorce I hated the next day. Then I would really be all alone.

I was sitting in the back of the courtroom as the two attorneys spoke quietly. I was so visibly upset that they decided not to have me testify before the judge. They knew how much I hated what was happening and were afraid of what this crazy man might say.

They were right. When the judge asked Maura if we had exhausted all possibilities to save the marriage, including counseling, she said yes, we had. I wanted to tell the judge that was a big lie. I had wanted professional marriage counseling, but she wouldn't go.

When Maura stepped down from the witness stand, I felt so all alone. I was just run over by a cement truck, and I had no one to help me get up.

Chapter 13

Just before I moved out, I began my role as a spokesperson for the mentally ill. Three days after one of my visits to the psych ward at Rush University Medical Center someone was knocking on my front door. It was Monday December 13, 1999 about 6 p.m. Neither Maura nor I was expecting company.

The young man had a camera around his neck. He identified himself as a photographer from the *Chicago Sun Times*. He said he wanted to take a picture of me for the next day's edition. We invited him in just before the phone rang. Reporter Maureen O'Donnell wanted to interview me as an example of someone who was getting treatment for his mental illness. US Surgeon General David Satcher had just released the first ever report by any US Surgeon General on mental illnesses. O'Donnell had called my boss, the president of the Mental Health Association of Illinois, looking for someone with a mental illness she could interview.

The following day the extra-large headline on the top of the front page read, "Mental Illness Ignored." Then the article:

One in five Americans suffer from a mental disorder, and nearly half of those with a severe mental illness fail to seek treatment, according to a historic report issued Monday by the US Surgeon General.

People often don't get help because of the stigma associated with mental illness, financial barriers or insurance problems, according to the report.

Mental disorders are not character flaws but are legitimate illnesses that respond to specific treatments, just as other health conditions respond to medical interventions.

Society can no longer afford to view mental health as separate and unequal to general health.

"My message to Americans is this," said Satcher, "if you, or a loved one, are experiencing what you believe might be the symptoms of a mental disorder, do not hesitate to seek effective treatment now."

Barrington resident Tom Ricke, who suffers from bipolar illness or manic depression, said treatment can make a difference.

"I've gotten literally more than 200 electric shock treatments, and they have helped me. I take a bunch of different medications and I see a doctor frequently," he said.

"I've also had to be hospitalized several times. Sometimes for long periods. The result of getting all this treatment and all of this care is I'm functioning. I am working at the Mental Health Association in Illinois where I'm doing some good. I don't know what would become of me if I wasn't getting the care I'm getting."

The document is a review of 3,000 academic studies and is the first and only report on mental health by a US Surgeon General.

Its effect on public awareness may rival that of the landmark 1964 Surgeon General's report on smoking and illness, mental health advocates said.

"We hope it will stimulate a lot of discussion," said Dr. Steven Potsic, Midwest administrator for the US Department of Health and Human Services.

"A decade or two ago, if you had cancer, that stigmatized the patient and families. Many times people didn't socialize with people with cancer. That has changed today."

"The country's top medical officer is coming out to talk about a problem which really is a health crisis," said the executive director of the Mental Health Association in Illinois, where Ricke is director of public education and communications. Ricke held high power jobs before "mental illness got the best of me," he said, including as a reporter for the *Detroit Free Press*, an editorial writer for the *New York Daily News*, chief speech writer for New York governor, Hugh Carey, director of corporate communications for Philip Morris and senior Vice President of Kraft.

Despite his efforts, "mental illness has totally ruined my life. I'm struggling to do the best I can. Five years ago, I had a teenage son who had the same mental illness I do, manic depression, and he committed suicide. Right now I'm going through the breakup of my marriage."

Based on the national estimate that mental disorders affect one in five Americans nationally, about two million Illinois residents are affected. A mental disorder is characterized by changes in thinking, mood and behavior.

About 500,000 state residents have a serious mental illness, Potsic said, such as schizophrenia, depression and anxiety disorders.

"To a great extent we are dumping our mental health problems on the streets of America," Satcher said in an interview.

"African Americans are less likely to get outpatient mental health services," Satcher said, "but are more likely to end up institutionalized, suggesting they are missing opportunities for early care."

That article started a trend with Chicago-area media. Whenever there was a relatively important story about mental illness and reporters were looking for an interview with a quotable patient, they would often call MHAI and ask for me.

For example, when a Houston-based company, Cyberonics, Inc., introduced a new hopeful device to treat really bad depression, I was called for an interview with two major newspapers and two local television stations.

A photographer came to my house again. This time the picture was for the *Daily Herald*, a large daily which covered the Chicago suburbs.

The device was called the Neuro-Cybernetic Prosthesis and was essentially a "pacemaker for the brain." A device about the size of a pocket watch was surgically implanted in a patient's chest. It was a generator/battery attached to the left vagus nerve by a very thin wire that sent regular small electrical impulses to the brain. The vagus nerve is a major pathway to the brain which is believed to help regulate mood. Stimulating this nerve has shown an increase in blood flow in areas of the brain associated with depression.

The device was to be tested in twenty US sites under FDA supervision to see if it could successfully treat patients with severe untreatable depression.

It is estimated that there are 1.2 million Americans who could have benefited from the device. Rush University Medical Center was the Chicago-based hospital chosen to test the new treatment.

The *Daily Herald's* story about the hopeful new treatment started with this description of my difficult-to-treat bipolar depression:

While other suburban commuters on the train checked stock prices or read e-mail on their laptop computers, Tom Ricke typed suicide notes.

"I've got a whole computer full of them," said Ricke, a 54-year-old Palatine man suffering from bipolar disorder, or manic depression. Ricke's life hasn't been an easy one.

A former political speech writer and corporate executive, Ricke now works part-time and collects disability. Last year, he and his wife of twenty-three years divorced. Six years ago, Ricke's sixteen-year-old son, also bipolar, killed himself. "This illness ruined my life," Ricke said. He's tried just about every treatment out there. Psychotherapy, pills. More pills.

"I've taken literally nearly every psychiatric medicine there is," he said. "I'll take it and it will work for a while. Then it will stop working and I'm back in the hospital, starting all over again."

He's even resorted to electric shock treatments in which doctors pass electrical current through the brain to induce seizures and bolster mood.

His 200 shock treatments have helped him some but there are

times when Ricke still grapples with mind-numbing bouts of depression. "I'll try anything," he said.

The *Daily Herald* article went on to describe how the new treatment is supposed to work with short interviews with patients who participated in the first pilot test of the device.

It stated that the treatment would cost about $20,000 a patient but predicted insurance companies would cover it. The article pointed out use of the device really isn't that expensive when compared to multiple shock treatments and the newer psychiatric prescription drugs.

The *Chicago Tribune* ran a similar article. After describing how the treatment is supposed to work and quoting professors from Harvard Medical School and Duke University Medical Center about how much the new treatment is needed, the article ran a few paragraphs about my experience with electric shock treatments:

Another drawback to shock therapy is that is produces short-term memory loss—or in the case of Palatine resident Tom Ricke after more than 200 treatments, what he describes as permanent memory loss.

"I hated getting the shock treatments," said Ricke, 53.

After nine years of fighting severe depression, Ricke has found some stability through a combination of medications and a history of shock treatments. But with his condition, he never knows how long the stability will last. As for the experimental therapy being tested in Chicago, Ricke said that if he takes a downturn again, "I'll try anything that works. I'd consider anything if it will help me."

I was also interviewed by reporters from two local television stations when I was working at the Mental Health Association in Illinois that day.

Three weeks after the announcement I met with the doctor at Rush University Medical Center who was in charge of the clinical trial. He told me I might be a good candidate for the experiment.

I cried while I told him about my stubborn bipolar depression and how I felt so hopeless and helpless in dealing with the horrific inner pain it caused. If there was a good chance this new device would help me, I was more than willing to take it.

It turned out that I could not be a candidate for the study because it dealt with only unipolar depression, not manic depression.

In the end, the pacemaker for the brain did not perform well during the national study and was not approved by the FDA.

Every year the Daily Herald puts out a special section on mental illnesses. Working closely with the Herald's editorial staff, I represented MHAI in the preparation of articles for the annual effort providing guidance about current mental health issues.

I wrote some of the editorial content. Advertising from pharmaceutical companies and local mental health care givers made the section profitable.

One long article I wrote described my fall from corporate America and the painful loss of my son, my career, my marriage, and my ability to function normally. I described how I was missing everything important in my life except my daughter Marie. I ended the article with a description of what I did to recover from the terrible symptoms of severe mental illness.

"The key to my progress is that I grasped onto whatever help there was and never let go. No matter how sick I was, I tried to stay determined to get better. I never gave up totally. Medicine, self-help groups, therapy with a psychologist and psychiatrist, multiple hospitalizations, ECT—they were all instrumental in my ongoing recovery. But, in the end, the crucial factor was my determination. In the end, my heart and soul won control over my mind and body.

"I am not cured. My mental illness limits what I can do. I still have episodes that require hospitalization. But I am better than I used to be. I am making progress.

"An important part of that progress is that I am working part-time for the Mental Health Association in Illinois where I am a member of a team that helps people with mental illness and their families."

In addition to being interviewed in the media and writing for the media, I became involved in Illinois politics by giving testimony about mental health insurance parity to the Illinois Insurance Committee.

The first time I testified was at a hearing in suburban Chicago. I told the legislators Mark's story. I told them how Mark used up all the insurance coverage for his illness, which had a lifetime cap of $15,000. He had two hospitalizations and was involved in group therapy, which seemed to help him. Then the insurance ran out and the support group "kicked him out." Months later I found Mark hanging in his bedroom closet.

Mark never mentioned suicide to anyone before he took his life. Of course we would have found a way to pay for the support group ourselves if we had any idea he was that ill. But it would have been better if our health insurance covered his mental illness with the same level of benefits that it had for all other illnesses.

"I'm not saying Mark would certainly still be alive if we had insurance parity," I told the committee, "but I believe that if there had been insurance parity for Mark's deadly bipolar disorder, it would have made a difference."

There were at least a hundred people at the hearing including a Barrington woman, who testified about losing her son who suffered from paranoid schizophrenia.

She found him dead in his bedroom after he committed suicide. His mental illnesses coverage had long reached its limit and his parents were doing the best they could to pay for his medical treatment anyway.

"I think it is a crime for lives to be lost and families to be discriminated against because of stigma and ignorance," she said.

Not everyone at the hearing was in favor of health insurance parity. The Illinois Chamber of Commerce said it was representing the state's business community in opposing health insurance parity. A spokesman for the Chamber said parity would just be too costly for employers. He told the committee that businesses at a minimum would have to cut both dental and eye care to afford mental illness insurance parity.

At least one company, First National Bank of Chicago, was

happy it expanded the range of mental health services covered by its insurance.

"It's not true parity, but it's close," said Dr. Dan Conti, director of employee assistance programs at the bank. For example, the bank's insurance covers 85 percent of the costs for the first twelve psychotherapy sessions. The rest are covered at 50 percent. The company also has a $2 million cap on all of its medical coverage which includes mental health services."

The hearing was covered by the media. For instance, the *Daily Herald* ran an article about the event. The first half of the article told Mark's story about how he died after losing his mental health insurance coverage.

Six months later I was asked to testify again at the final state legislative hearing on a specific proposed parity law. My boss didn't think I could navigate the trip by myself, so she encouraged me to go with a woman I was dating at the time. We drove to Springfield the night before the hearing. I had decided to use my testimony to point out that mental illnesses can be just as fatal as other illnesses and therefore deserves the same health insurance coverage.

I began my testimony by introducing myself and telling them how mental illness had ruined my life. I told them how close I had come to dying from suicide. I told them about my hospitalizations, about all of the ECT I had received and all of the medications I still took. I did my best to explain that mental Illnesses were medical illnesses of the brain, illnesses that could be just as damaging and fatal as other medical illnesses. Then I told them Mark's story. There was a collective gasp from the audience when I talked about how he died after losing insurance coverage for his illness.

"If you remember anything I tell you today, I hope it is this," I said. "Mental illness is not just patients' difficult struggles with mood, speech, and behavior. It is life and death. Untreated bipolar disorder kills twenty percent of its patients by suicide. Other major mental illnesses kill as many as ten to even fifteen percent of their patients. Tremendous pain and suffering, life and death. How can anyone say that people with mental illnesses don't deserve medical treatment?"

The part-time lobbyist who the mental health organizations were using came up to me and said, "You hit it out of the park."

That parity law won legislative approval, but it was a very limited parity, not covering at least seventy percent of state businesses. MHAI still considered it a significant victory. You had to start somewhere. Years later Obamacare would eventually make health insurance parity the law of the land.

The National Mental Health Association started a political program called the Voter Empowerment Project.

The idea was to get mentally ill people and their friends and relatives to become aware of political issues that affect them. There were two parts to the program. The first was to get people with mental illnesses and their families registered to vote.

The next step was to educate them on government/political issues that had an effect on their lives. Some of the issues included persistent annual cuts to state and local mental health services despite the obvious growing need for the services. State mental hospitals and urban mental health clinics had a difficult time with funding even when Illinois and Chicago were not broke. Now the state is billions in debt and the city of Chicago owes hundreds of millions.

Mental health services didn't stand a chance of avoiding annual cuts.

Busy mental health clinics in Chicago have been closed. Over the years a number of state mental hospitals have been shut down. The remaining hospitals close a number of their beds every year because of budget cuts.

Now some people who have no health insurance and need state mental health services cannot be admitted to state hospitals because there is no room for them.

Before psychotropic drugs became available in the late fifties people with serious mental Illnesses were warehoused in large state institutions where there was little hope of recovery. Then new medicines treated some of the obvious symptoms of certain mental illnesses and gave caregivers reason to release them back into the community.

The theory was people taking medications that altered brain chemistry and lessened the symptoms of mental illnesses would be treated much better in their communities than in state institutions. The problem wasn't the theory. The community-based treatment didn't work for those who really needed it because it was never properly funded.

In the earlier days of large state institutions, patients at Elgin State Hospital actually worked a farm that provided some of their food. Decades later medicated patients who were considered well enough to leave the hospital were bussed to a specific street corner in the uptown neighborhood of Chicago. They carried a suitcase and a small amount of money. They were really all on their own.

Today there are two totally different worlds for people with mental illnesses.

I have been very fortunate to have some of the best possible treatment.

Unfortunately, I believe those of us who are getting effective treatment are still in the minority. A large part of the homeless who beg on street corners and roam urban areas are people with untreated mental illnesses. Jails house more mentally ill people than any other institutions.

For example, the LA County jail and the Cook County jail in Chicago each house more people with mental illnesses than any private or public mental health institution in America. The majority of the mentally ill in jails are locked up for rather minor offenses and cannot pay their bail.

There was plenty of room for dramatic improvement of government mental health policy and programs. The Mental Health Association in Illinois, along with other local mental health advocate groups, started their own statewide voter empowerment program.

They wanted to be able to claim that the program was run by people with mental illnesses, so I was named chairman of the effort.

After the first several meetings we put together a six-page pamphlet aimed at people with mental illnesses and their families. It reminded our members that we still "endure a horrible stigma; suffer personal and institutional discrimination; face a society that blames us more than it helps us and know that government too often turns its back on us."

The pamphlet went on to say that voting for candidates "who take the needs of people with mental illness seriously" can make a significant difference in how we are treated.

It promised to have political office holders and candidates fill out questionnaires about mental health issues and then share the information with the mental health community. It also said we would provide the names and addresses of politicians and office holders so our members could let them know our positions on mental health issues.

We offered help registering voters and helping them get to the polls on election day. The brochure had a tear-out section asking for the name, email address, street address, and phone number of the "mental health consumer." The brochure had our address and a postage-paid number on it so that the information would be mailed to us.

I attended at least three gatherings of people with mental illnesses where we handed out the brochures and explained the program. We received many postcards in the mail, but we were unable to follow up.

MHAI and the other organizations behind the program were not-for-profit agencies that depended on contributions for all of their activities. Psychiatric medications are one of the most profitable medicines offered by the pharmaceutical industry. The drug companies were the primary funders of mental health organizations. MHAI also received funds for specific programs from state government agencies, but there were no funds earmarked for the state voter-empowerment project at the nonprofit agencies that started it. We tried to get funding for the effort from our traditional supporters, but they were not interested.

The program died from lack of financial support before it was able to reach a significant number of people with mental illnesses and their families. During the start-up of the Illinois program we learned that it would have been very challenging and difficult for it to work even if it had been fully funded. Because of the stigma and shame associated with mental illnesses, it seemed like a good number of patients and their families were uncomfortable with the prospect of bringing public attention to their treatment and funding issues.

In order to obtain and keep its license for broadcasting, Chicago cable television had to make a special channel for public service. Much of the programming on that channel was devoted to non-profit agencies. We applied for our opportunity for this free publicity and were granted a half hour each week on Thursdays at 4 p.m.

All of the non-profit programming had to be call-in shows where the audience could call a special number and get answers to their questions live on TV.

Putting on a show took at least three people—the moderator, the guest, and a person to screen phone calls.

In addition to being the moderator, I had to book guests for the show. The program ran for two eight-week seasons. I was amazed at the power of television, even this small cable TV show. Just about everyone I asked was able to be a guest. Prominent psychiatrists and psychologists changed their patient schedules in order to appear on the program. I was able to book attorneys and legislators who were experts in mental health issues. I also had leaders in non-profit mental health agencies.

The guest and I sat in two chairs that were so close they touched one another. There was a table in front of us and a large sign in back of us that spelled out Mental Health Association in Illinois and gave the phone number for call-ins. The television camera was in a fixed position in front of us.

For the first few programs I had a hard time looking straight into the camera. I had become so shy I rarely could look someone in the eye. I looked down or around. It was a symptom of my illness and/or the medications I was taking.

After I made myself look into the camera, I thought I was a good host who asked the right questions and elicited interesting answers from my guests. Friends who watched the programs later told me I was still obviously nervous. They said I was moving my head back and forth and letting my hands shake in front of the camera. They also said I talked too fast, but I got a little better after each show.

We talked about why so many people with mental illnesses end up begging on the streets where jail can seem like a blessing because it offers shelter and three meals a day. We discussed pending legislation involving people with mental illnesses. Doctors answered questions about specific illnesses and the treatment for them.

We discussed the fact that there were few public programs to make mental health services available to the fifty percent of people with mental illnesses who according to the US Surgeon General were receiving absolutely no mental health care. I don't think there ever was any public service advertising about anything to do with mental illnesses.

I knew enough about mental illness issues that I was prepared to answer some of the questions myself. I had my daughter Marie as a guest. She had been so supportive to me over the years I thought her interview would benefit friends and relatives of people with mental illnesses by showing them how important their support could be in a patient's recovery from mental illness.

In her emotional interview, she told the audience how difficult it was for her to grow up with a mentally ill brother who killed himself.

She was on the verge of weeping when she spoke about me and my history of severe mental illness with strong suicidal behavior. She never gave up on me no matter how I behaved. She said she was proud of me for how I never quit fighting the illness.

Tears fell down my face as she talked about what it was like to have a father who didn't get up and go to work each day like all her friends' fathers. She didn't talk about how I tormented her with my suicide threats.

I would call her to say goodbye when I was overcome with suicidal thoughts. I would say how much I loved her and then tell her I would soon die and then hang up the phone so she couldn't try to talk me out of it. She got to the point where she became so upset with my dark threats, she screened my calls and wouldn't answer them, so I would leave her dark messages of utter despair and hopelessness. I would say that I was going to do what was best for me. I would tell her it wasn't her fault and that I loved her more than I could express.

Marie felt like I was putting my life in her hands and she was petrified of talking with me fearing she would say something that would somehow encourage my longing for death.

Once in a while when she did take my calls, I would talk to her. I would say goodbye and then hang up the phone before she could reply.

She didn't know what she could do to help me because I wouldn't let her interfere with my suicidal behavior. She would cry and cry after my selfish phone calls. She felt so sad and helpless.

Memories of Mark's successful suicide savaged her heart. She would call emergency rooms of local hospitals to see if I was there and still alive. She worked part-time at a Starbucks when she was in college. One day after a terrible goodbye call from me she hid in the backroom of the store and wept uncontrollably for more than an hour.

Since she was the only supervisor there that afternoon, she had to finish her shift. The tears slowly ran down her face for the rest of the afternoon. Her terrible sorrow and fear lasted long after I hung up the phone. Whenever she thought of me, she feared she would lose me like she lost Mark whose death changed her life so dramatically.

Some of the students called her the "suicide girl" when she attended the same high school as Mark.

She became involved with several after-school activities in hopes fellow students would associate her with these endeavors more than Mark's death.

She was involved with the school's drama program where she

would have important roles in their plays. She was a member of the renowned Barrington's Children's Choir where her featured voice was appreciated. In addition to Chicago area concerts, the choir sang at Carnage Hall in New York City and in a London concert hall.

When she felt really bad, she would run and run around the school grounds until she felt a little better.

While she was busy with these after-school activities, she also got nearly all A's in her classes. Another big reason she stayed away from her home as long as she could was to escape the bitter fighting between Maura and me as we headed for an emotional and painful divorce. I was so scared of ending up alone with no one to help care for me when the illness took over.

Marie and I ended up in Dr. Francis's office where we had a serious discussion about my calling and emailing Marie with my suicidal rants.

Marie cried when she told me how much my suicidal communications hurt and scared her. She and Dr. Francis asked me to remember how much terrible pain Mark's death caused me.

They explained my suicidal threats caused Marie the same type of horrible pain we experienced at Mark's passing. She lost her brother to suicide. Now she would lose her father the same way and there was nothing she could do about it. She felt so helpless.

I came so close to taking my life. She just knew my ongoing suicidal behavior would eventually be successful. She could not imagine the permanent horror of losing both her father and her brother to manic depression's fatal symptom.

I thought my suicide calls to Marie were to tell her how much I loved her before I died. During the session with Dr. Francis I began to realize how I was hurting her with these calls.

"What am I supposed to do? What t can I do when you call me to tell me you are going to kill yourself?" she said.

I felt the pain in her heart about my suicidal ravings.

I felt so bad as I compared my feelings about Mark's death to her feelings about mine. Maura ran away from me. Marie loved and supported me no matter how mentally ill I was. And what did I do? I tortured her with my suicidal madness.

The one-hour session turned out to be a miracle of sorts. Suicide still haunted me from time to time, but I never called Marie again with suicidal goodbyes.

Chapter 14

After I finally moved out to my apartment, my suicidal urges came with me. My health professionals and my family were convinced that I would have to live in an institution to save my life. Dr. Francis thought she would never see me again. Dr. Easton wanted me to continue the shock treatments hoping they would finally quiet the suicidal screaming in my brain.

I surprised everyone, especially me, when I actually improved slowly after leaving Maura and her painful rejections of my affection and friendship. Living in an apartment all by myself was dark and quiet torture. I had no real friends. I didn't know what to do on the days I didn't commute downtown to work at the mental health association. There was a Blockbuster Video store nearby and I rented at least four movies a week.

I tried to meet someone by using online dating services. I knew some women would dump me after they discovered I was mentally ill. The more time I spent with them before I told them about my illness, the harder it would be on me when they decided to walk away. So I told my dates I was bipolar soon after we met and before I could develop romantic feelings. Needless to say, I had mostly one-date relationships.

I was very sad and lonely. When my bipolar depression kicked in, the suicidal urges and thoughts tried to take over my mind. It would be one certain way to end my bipolar pain. When I wasn't depressed, I was numb. The medicine I took did a better job restraining my manic side than arresting my deeply sad depression. Numb was okay. It sure beat suicidal ideation.

I spent a lot of time in my apartment. It had two bedrooms. I used the smaller one as an office. The living room was large enough for a couch, love seat, coffee and end tables, and a large bookcase that held a rather old-fashioned stereo and television.

There was a dining area with a wooden floor next to the living room. It was big enough for a large dining room set and china cabinet. I rarely ate there. I preferred to eat off the coffee table where I would watch TV.

The kitchen was small. It had minimal cabinet space. There was one small counter next to the sink where I used my microwave. The refrigerator, stove, and dishwasher had to be at least ten to fifteen years old. I lived on frozen dinners cooked in the microwave. The only time I used the stove was to cook Thanksgiving dinner with Marie. During nice weather I occasionally cooked on a gas grill on my patio off of the living room. I didn't do this very often. Who wants to barbecue for one person? For that matter, who wants to cook only for themselves? I had a hard time adjusting to a one-person life.

When Maura and I were together we went to church on Sundays with the children. Then we would go out for breakfast afterward. I wouldn't go to church or out to eat by myself.

I wouldn't go to movies by myself. I wanted to avoid feeling so alone where couples, families, and groups of friends filled up nearly all of the places. It made me feel there was something very wrong with me that made it so hard to find friends to share these activities.

Although I felt that way, I wasn't totally alone. I could talk to my boss at the Mental Health Association. She and I often took the same train downtown to work.

I began to attend dual-diagnosis meetings where mentally ill people with drinking issues held meetings just like Alcoholics

Anonymous meetings. These twelve-step gatherings took place on Saturday mornings, and a group of us always went to lunch afterward. So I had opportunities to interact with others three to four days a week. I was still very lonely.

I missed the intellectual intimacy of a close friendship, and I longed for the closeness of a woman. I learned the hard way that you could still feel all alone with other people, but I didn't stop trying to make it better.

I met Margaret at a weekend singles dance at the Barn of Barrington where middle-aged men and women looked for companionship. She was a couple of years older than me. We danced a few times and shared phone numbers before we left. She was attractive and seemed intelligent. I told myself I could do much worse.

We dated for more than a year. Even though we had little in common we got along most of the time, but not all of the time. Sometimes when I would do or say something she didn't like she would say our relationship was over. She would leave me alone, but the separations never lasted more than a week or two. I would always apologize for whatever was bothering her at the time, and she would take me back. I was terrified of losing her and being all alone again.

I was still receiving electric shock treatments when we met. Like most people, Margaret lacked an understanding of mental illness. I was surprised when she didn't react much to my situation when I told her I was bipolar. After I was with her and went through about a dozen shock treatments, she called Dr. Easton and told him she didn't think I still needed them anymore. After two or three more, he stopped them. I haven't had one since, but I still wrestled with suicide.

I told Margaret about Mark's death and explained that I still had to fight strong suicidal urges. After our relationship blossomed into some mutual affection, I did call her at least a couple of times with explanations of why I had to kill myself.

I don't know if I called asking for help or just to say goodbye. One time she raced the fifteen miles to my apartment hoping she would arrive in time to save me. Another time she took me to a Catholic service I had never heard of. It was called a healing service.

The people who wanted to be healed lined up at the communion rail as a priest who was known for his healing powers walked from person to person saying special prayers and putting holy oils on their foreheads. After he finished with each person, the men and women who received the healing treatment fell back. A group of volunteers who were called "catchers" caught the people on their way to the ground.

Margaret knew a masseuse and hoped that getting a professional massage would help my depression. The massage felt great, but the forlorn sadness was still there when it was over.

Another time when I was down and dismal and starting to yield to the suicidal commands, she took me to a priest she knew at 11 p.m. on a weeknight. I explained to the priest that I was bipolar and felt like I was losing my ongoing battle with suicide.

Margaret told the priest I was spiritually bankrupt and in need of God's grace. She spoke as if I could be well if I really wanted to. She complained about how I treated her in general, telling the priest I was cruel and insensitive. I think she was hoping the priest would chastise me for how she claimed I wronged her and then say special prayers for a spiritual cure.

The priest told us he would keep us in his prayers and then told Margaret that I did suffer from a medical condition that required a doctor's care. He urged me to pray for God's help, and he told Margaret that her kindness and understanding would certainly help me more than her criticism.

The priest's prayers may have helped. I did get better after our session. The commands became more quiet urges. I continued to take my prescriptions and see Dr. Francis and Dr. Easton.

In a few weeks the suicidal delusions stopped, and I was a free man for several months.

Margaret and I took a trip to Lake Tahoe. My sister, Peggy, and my parents lived in Sacramento which is about a full day's drive from the famous lake. They met us at the hotel we were staying in. That night we went on a dinner cruise. The food was very good. The scenery was fantastic. There I was with four people who loved me and wanted the best for me. Despite everything that should have made me happy, I felt devastated. While they were still eating dinner, I got up and walked over to the boat's railing. I stood there staring at the dark water below. It took every bit of willpower I had to not jump in.

Peggy sensed something was wrong. She stood up and walked over to where I was clinging to the rail. She took me by the arm and gently pulled me back to the table. I rarely cry, but that night tears rolled down my cheeks. The profound sadness came out of nowhere, but it only lasted for a day or two.

From time to time Margaret's emotionally insecure behavior made me think I should leave her, but I was too afraid of the loneliness that could bring back my suicidal longings.

One Saturday afternoon she was looking around in my walk-in closet and discovered a huge four-by-three foot portrait of Maura, me, and the children. We had the picture taken by a professional photographer when everything in our lives was very good. It was a sunny day in our backyard. We all were smiling brilliantly. I could not hang it on the wall because of the terrible loss I felt looking at it. So I hid it in that closet where an occasional glance didn't hurt so much.

Margaret was furious. She was so upset she yelled and screamed and threatened to leave me. I could tell she meant it. She really scared me.

In her mind the fact I kept the picture and didn't throw it away meant I still loved Maura and my former family more than her.

As she put on her coat to leave forever, I grabbed the picture out of the closet. I broke the wooden frame to pieces and ripped the photo to shreds as I stood in front of her. As I took the portrait's remains to the outside garbage bin, she took off her coat. She didn't leave me, but she was cold and distant the rest of the weekend. From that day on I have missed the ability to glance at the happiest time in my life. The irrational, overwhelming fear of living all alone again fueled my bipolar illness and made me destroy the photo. Today I can't believe I did it.

For the next several months we grew closer together. We talked about our past and hopes for our future. We were intimate. We had fun. From time to time she was still critical of me, but I learned to ignore it. It was just Margaret being Margaret I told myself.

We were going out for dinner on a Saturday night. I could tell something was really bothering her. After dinner when we were waiting for desert, she asked me if Marie was pregnant. I told her no.

Then she told me that one of her girlfriends warned her about me and Marie. The woman told Margaret that she thought her former male lover wanted to have sex with his own daughter. In the past I tried to help Margaret understand how much I loved Marie. I recall telling her that I loved Marie "ferociously." Margaret didn't have any children and didn't understand the special love parents have for their children. She warned me to stop being too close to Marie.

I could not believe what I was hearing. As she continued to talk to me as if I wanted to be intimate with Marie, I realized I could no longer have a relationship with Margaret.

It took a couple of weeks for me to tell her I was leaving. I was still afraid of being all alone again, but there was no way I could remain close to a woman who worried that I was sleeping with my daughter. When I left her at her condo, she wept and begged me not to go. I didn't turn back to look at her. I couldn't wait to get out of there. This made me realize there are some situations much worse than being alone.

Chapter 15

My troubles with the Mental Health Association of Illinois and my boss started at a cocktail party fundraiser.

I was keeping an eye on two video players that were showing tapes of my TV shows. As I tried to mingle, my boss approached me with a man she had been talking to for a good while. He was a bank executive who worked with non-profit agencies, and she had added him to our board of directors. She introduced us by saying we probably had a lot in common because we were both raised in Detroit.

That turned out to be quite an understatement. Bob and I had actually attended the same Jesuit high school and college around the same time. We agreed to have lunch sometime soon.

When we met a few weeks later we talked for a long time. After we shared some of our experiences growing up in the Motor City, our conversation turned to what was going on at the mental health association.

I let my guard down and shared my real feelings about how our association was not fulfilling its mission to help people with mental illnesses. I explained that a non-profit agency had to develop programs that would attract the interest of potential sponsors. To survive you have to go where the money is. So MHAI developed and staffed programs to lessen bullying in schools. We ran a program that trained teachers and parents to help students deal with tragedies such as school shootings and the death of teachers or parents. These programs were certainly worthwhile, but they did not have much to do with helping people with basic mental illnesses. I told him I thought MHAI could become a real leader in dealing with topical mental health issues.

In the distant past, MHAI conducted annual reports on the quality of care in state mental health hospitals. The hospitals received grades for their performance in several categories.

I told him about some of the ideas I had discussed with my boss that were going nowhere. For example, what about a symposium on how the Cook County jail can improve services for the prisoners who are mentally ill? Most of these prisoners are charged with relatively minor crimes. There are always more of them in the winter when being in jail at least provides protection from the cold weather, a place to sleep, and three meals a day. The county sheriff responsible for mentally ill prisoners was saying that many of them needed special care not available in the criminal justice/jail system.

So why not bring together experts in mental health and law enforcement to discuss the problems of having so many mentally ill prisoners in the Cook County jail? The media would cover the gathering. The group would issue a final report that would offer the experts' suggestions on how to improve conditions for mentally ill prisoners. The in-depth report would focus on specific programs and services that would serve both the interests of the jail and its mentally ill inmates. It would also describe the horrible existence of the mentally ill people left to beg on the streets before they get to the jail. How annual cuts of city and state mental health services are responsible for the lack of necessary mental health care in our communities would also be a subject covered in the report.

All of the media coverage would mention the fact that MHAI conducted the symposium and issued the report of its findings. This would improve MHAI's reputation and increase its ability to raise funds. More important, it could end up providing some help for the fifty percent of mentally ill people not receiving any professional services.

Bob agreed with what I had to say and told me there were several members of the board of directors who felt the same way.

It made me feel like a traitor, but I offered him a copy of a memo I had sent to my boss with my ideas for how MHAI could better serve mentally ill people by focusing on issues that could improve the quality of care available to them.

After I sent it to him I decided I didn't want to be disloyal to my boss, so I told her about our conversation about the group of board members interested in changing the focus of the agency's efforts. I didn't know it at the time, but she was very aware of this.

In the meantime, I thought I was doing quite well with the TV show. I also asked Kay Jamison to accept a special award from us and speak at our annual fundraising lunch.

Even though her husband was extremely ill, she agreed to travel from her home in Washington, DC, to Chicago where she gave a speech about some of the issues covered in her best-selling book, *An Unquiet Mind*. The memoir focuses on Kay's personal struggles with manic depression and suicide. It is one of several books she has written on mental illness issues including *Night Falls Fast*, a book about suicide. The professor from Johns Hopkins University has also co-authored the medical textbook on manic depression. She has received many honors and awards for her work and is a true national leader in the field of mental health. The luncheon was a terrific success. It sold out soon after her appearance was announced. On the way back to the airport she agreed to help me with this book.

That was several years ago and I haven't been able to get back in touch with her since.

It's taken me many years to get this far. I have had to overcome a tremendous fear of what my friends and relatives—especially Marie—would think of me after reading about the abhorrent behavior that I now believe was shaped by my manic depression. MHAI's board of directors was appreciative of my work on the successful luncheon and my work on the television shows, but they had serious misgivings about keeping me on the payroll.

I was only being paid about $600 a month which used to be the limit you could earn and still receive Social Security disability benefits including Medicare. As the amount you could earn and still receive disability benefits was increased, I asked MHAI to raise my pay to meet the limit.

They refused. The board claimed that MHAI could not afford to pay me a couple of hundred more a month. Since my work was not paid by any grants, I was overhead for MHAI.

A few months after the luncheon the chairwoman of the board of directors fired me. The association simply couldn't afford to pay me anymore. I was enraged. I stood up and told her off. I slammed the door on my way out.

After I calmed down a bit, I realized I was only half done with the second season of the television show. I asked my boss to let me finish the season. I would work from home and come in on Thursdays when the show aired. She agreed and I finished the season without being paid.

Several months later my boss left MHAI to work for a large pharmaceutical company. Her new job was perfect for her. She managed the drug company's financial support of non-profit associations like MHAI in three or four Midwestern states. From what I have heard she really liked corporate life and was doing quite well.

After I left MHAI I had to endure another terrible loneliness. Every empty day and night increased my suffering and fueled my deep bipolar depression.

When the mania took the driver's seat, it wasn't a happy energy or fun high. It was a desperately sad and painful combination of bipolar mania and depression called a mixed state or dysphoric mania. The depression made me think of suicide, and the sharp mania offered the energy to do it.

During this time, I met a man named Harry, and we became friends. My life got a little better thanks to this friendship. We would go to lunch every couple of weeks. We played golf once in a while. He told me he didn't have a lot of friends, and he appreciated our friendship. I really liked him. He had an outgoing personality and a great sense of humor, but he eventually took advantage of me when I was still fighting my bipolar illness.

Harry offered me his services as a financial advisor. I still had some funds left over from my share of the Kraft settlement. It wasn't a big amount since Maura got half as a result of the divorce; it was all I had and mitigated my inability to work full-time at any meaningful job.

I thought Harry would look at my assets and offer a variety of options for their growth. Instead he advised me to put the entire amount into annuities. It turns out he was working solely for Alliance, a company that specialized in annuities. Instead of diversifying my investments in a variety of programs such as mutual funds and stocks, I followed Harry's advice and put it all in three different annuities.

Harry received a commission from these investments, but I didn't mind this at the time. I trusted him and valued his friendship. The returns were about average for the first few years. The concept was I would receive a monthly payment from one annuity while the other two grew enough to cover those payments. It didn't exactly turn out that way, but I was satisfied with the results. After all, Harry was my good friend. He wouldn't hurt me financially. We maintained our friendship. I continued to trust him.

A couple of years after the initial investment in the annuities, Harry visited me in my apartment and told me he was now working with Fidelity. He said I should take my funds out of the annuities and give the money to him for investments in Fidelity programs. I was wrestling with my illness at the time and didn't want to lose Harry's friendship so I told him I would follow his advice. I signed something he would use to shut down the annuities. I found out later that there were some penalties for early termination of the annuities.

I knew Harry would get more commissions from the new investments, but I still trusted him and valued his friendship.

I had very little, if any, self-esteem. Time seemed to be in slow motion. I had no job, no place to go, nothing to do, just a couple of friends I saw occasionally. I continued my weekly sessions with Dr. Francis. I saw Dr. Easton every few weeks.

I took my meds as prescribed, but I was still very depressed. I still thought of suicide as a possible escape from the pain of my madness and its symptoms. Dr. Francis and I talked about the possibility of me volunteering somewhere as a way to get me out of my apartment and put some people in my life.

I went to the only place I knew had a volunteer program. It was Good Shepherd Hospital in Barrington which was a thirty-minute drive from my home. I did several jobs there. I visited patients bringing them water or a newspaper or my temporary company.

I also worked in the emergency room greeting patients as they arrived. I asked them to tell me their symptoms, and I would write them down and send them to see the triage nurse. The hardest part was trying to placate patients who didn't want to wait, even for a few minutes.

One man took a swing at me when I asked his wife about her symptoms. He was so upset with his wife's illness that a delay of even a couple of minutes was too much for him to bear. Fortunately, there wasn't a line to see the triage nurse, and there was an empty room for the couple. On his way out a few hours later the man apologized for his impatience.

Another time a man struggled to reach my desk, which was about sixty feet from the door. He was grey and fighting very hard to breathe. He was clutching his chest. It seemed to me he needed immediate attention. I took him to the triage nurse even though she was seeing someone else. She took one look at the man and rushed him in a wheelchair to the room equipped to handle heart attacks.

Later the nurse told me the man survived his heart attack and was resting upstairs in the intensive care unit. That made me happy, a feeling I had not experienced in a long time.

Volunteering was good for me. It got me out of my apartment a couple of days a week and gave me situations where I could be useful, but it didn't help pay the bills. My disability payments paid for the rent, but not much else. I looked in the newspaper and online to try to find part-time work. I had a few interviews, but nothing came of them.

One of the men attending our Saturday morning dual diagnosis meetings worked part-time for a local Sears-Kmart store. He knew I was looking for work, so he invited me to apply there. He was well-regarded, and his recommendation got me hired right away. It didn't pay much more than minimum wage, and since I only worked part-time, I didn't have to worry about earning more than my disability allowed.

I had a hard time working the cash register. I was just too slow, causing a frustrated line of people waiting for me. I watched the teens playing their cash registers like a piano. I felt old and decrepit. I felt slow and depressed. It seemed like there was either not much to do except stand there waiting for customers or checking out a long line of impatient customers waiting for my services. The smart shoppers noticed how slow I was and went to other cashiers.

After a few months the management there found a new place for me. Spring was coming and they needed someone to work in the garden center. I was to keep the place stocked with plants, flowers, and gardening equipment. I had to check people out on the cash register there, but the lines were never very long. I also had to sweep the floor. That was one of the lowest and most painful times I ever had to endure. The man who once was a senior vice president of Kraft foods who had been in the Oval Office visiting the President was now sweeping dirty floors in a Sears/Kmart store for not much more than minimum wage.

The personal and professional loss in my life would have been enough to make anybody depressed. I think it was worse for me because I suffered with bipolar illness.

I still shuffled my feet when walking. I lurched from side to side. I never looked anyone in the eye. Everything seemed to go in slow motion. Everything seemed painful. I couldn't wait to get back to my lonely apartment where I was used to my quiet solitude.

I continued to volunteer at Good Shepherd. I liked working there much better than working at Sears. I became friendly with the woman who managed the volunteer department. Probably because the hospital was located in the ultra-wealthy suburb of Barrington where wives and retired men didn't have to work and some teens were required to participate in some form of community service, there were more than 800 volunteers. Just about every department in the hospital had volunteers to help with the work load.

After several months of my volunteering, they offered me a paying job in the volunteer office. The opportunity was for a 4 to 8 p.m. shift Monday through Friday. I would mainly interact with teens who worked the after-school shift. They were having a hard time finding someone to work that shift. They had been staffing it with younger people who would not show up and/or quit after a few months. It paid more than my job at Sears but not quite enough to threaten my disability and Medicare. It would get me out of the house every weekday. It would put more people in my life, and, best of all, it came with good health insurance.

I decided to take the job although I had some real doubts about how I would function there. The hospital health insurance became my primary medical coverage and Medicare became my secondary insurance paying for what my hospital insurance didn't pay. The result was I hardly ever got a medical bill for any type of care from doctor visits, clinic appointments, medical tests, surgery, and hospital stays.

I had the first of three open-back surgeries while I worked at Good Shepherd Hospital.

I had them done by a surgeon at Rush University Medical Center, which is a major medical school and the hospital where I was admitted so many times for my psychiatric care and electric shock treatments.

The bills I received for all three surgeries, including presurgical workups and weeks in a rehab, totaled only about $3,000.

I did have to pay for a portion of my prescriptions that were only partially covered by Medicare. After some coverage I found myself in the "doughnut hole" where I had to pay nearly full price for the prescriptions for at least seven months. I used my Mastercard to help me manage.

I met Barbara online. On our first date I discovered she was pretty, smart, sexy, and had a great sense of humor. She was a partner in her own business, so I figured she must be financially independent. I was more attracted to her than to any other woman I met since breaking up with Maura, and the feeling seemed to be mutual.

Early on in the relationship, she told me about her horrible childhood. Both of her parents were severe alcoholics. Their lives made *The Days of Wine and Roses* look like a picnic. Barbara and her sister and brother would be left to fend for themselves for days at a time. She remembers how the other children made fun of her because she had to wear the same dress to school for more than a week. After Barbara's parents split up, Barbara's mother remarried another drinking partner she knew from her favorite bar. Her step-father didn't bother her or her sister, but the alcohol fueled neglect, and psychological torture of the children continued until they left home. Barbara's brother became a barely functioning alcoholic who always had a drink or can of beer in his hand. Her sister married a saintly man who took good care of her and their three sons.

Barbara seemed to have put those demons behind her. I didn't realize then that she did a terrific job of hiding the effects of her damaged childhood.

After she told me about her lost childhood, I wanted to dry her tears, put my arms around her, and tell her things would be all right.

She divorced her first husband claiming he didn't pay enough attention to her. I didn't want to make the same mistake.

We enjoyed a whirlwind romance right from the beginning. We saw each other at least twice a week. She was co-owner of an exercise club for women. She and her best friend wanted a Curves franchise, but none were available in their area.

So they bought a different franchise that was modeled after Curves. Every two or three hours starting at 6 a.m. women came in to exercise, making movements in a circle to lively music. The sessions lasted about half an hour.

Barbara's mother took a second mortgage on her house and gave the proceeds to Barbara for her share of the franchise costs. When I visited their store, they certainly weren't crowded, but they did have a group of about twenty regulars that was growing slowly despite the competition from local Curves franchises.

Barbara's partner did not quit her regular job, so Barbara staffed the program full-time. When school started in the fall, I volunteered to open the franchise each weekday morning so she could get her two girls off to school. It opened at 6 a.m., and I'm not usually a morning person, but I was never late. Early in the morning before work was the busiest time for the business. It was an all-women format and I could tell some of the participants were not comfortable with me. So I hid in the office most of the time avoiding the exercise area except when I had to change the music. I also collected fees from the customers.

Vivid memories of her childhood weren't the only thoughts that made Barbara cry. When she shared the more recent bad news with me, she wept so hard she could barely speak. She had secretly married a man she met when she was on vacation by herself. She began the affair with him before divorcing her first husband.

Barbara developed breast cancer, and her lover hung around to support her after she had a breast removed. She lost all of her hair to chemotherapy and had to wear a wig.

It was determined that she was cancer-free after her surgery.

After she divorced her children's father, she went on a trip with her new lover. They married at a local county clerk's office. They were having fun. Even though he moved in after they were married, Barbara didn't tell her children she was married to the new man in their house. She told her children, neighbors and some friends that her visitor was a friend who needed a place to stay so she agreed to have him stay for a while. The only people who knew she was married to her visitor were her mother and her best friend. He slept on the couch while Barbara slept with her younger daughter.

Her new husband wanted everyone to know they were married. Barbara didn't want anyone to know. One day when they were really screaming at each other he became violent with her. She took the children and put them in her car.

He'd stood in back of the car so she couldn't move it. They were still screaming at each other. He kept shouting "We're married. I'm your husband. You can't treat me like this." She told him she was taking the children and would not come back until he was gone.

Eventually some neighbors heard the commotion and came over to help Barbara. They held her husband while she moved the car out of the driveway. He packed his things and left the next day.

I suppose this story should have been a warning for me. Why was she going on vacation by herself? Why not vacation with her immediate family? Did her first husband really totally ignore her? Then there was all the sneaking around during the affair. She didn't seem to feel at all guilty for cheating on her first husband.

She didn't mind that her friends and neighbors knew she was living with another man, but she didn't want them to know she was married to him.

I didn't pay any attention to any of the obvious warning signals. It had been decades since I fooled around. Given my ancient history with women, who was I to judge Barbara?

I held her while she cried and felt very sorry for her that her second marriage was so screwed up. I saw her as a victim. I felt a huge wave of affection wash over me. I wanted our relationship to be so close, affectionate, and full of mutual understanding that it would make up for her childhood and the turmoil of her first two marriages. I wanted to make her happy. She deserved to be happy.

The romance was intoxicating for me. It had been many years since I had been happy with Maura, many years since I felt I had good reason to be really happy about anything.

Yes, I had experienced the manic side of bipolar disorder, but those highs were just not the same as the terrific feelings that mixed my madness with true mutual love.

At first Dr. Francis thought Barbara was good for me since I could use my experience with coping with symptoms of my mental illness to help her fight her demons.

I would actually be helping someone, and that would help my low self-esteem.

The oldest of Barbara's two daughters was just about to enter high school when I arrived on the scene. The younger daughter was in elementary school. Barbara and I often took walks around the neighborhood where we could talk without her children listening. When we were walking one weekend afternoon we were talking about finances, and I told her how much I was worth. I expected her to tell me she was worth more. After all, she was a partner in a new business. She must have some resources.

When she didn't respond, I just figured she was a private person not comfortable discussing her personal finances. I didn't know then that she was broke and that her mother had taken a second mortgage and given Barbara the money to purchase the business with her friend.

It turned out that all she had was a pile of unpaid bills. Even if I had known that, it wouldn't have made a difference. I seemed to be in love no matter what she told me about her past. She was the victim of cruel circumstances. She could do no wrong.

On our next walk around the block the following day, I asked her to marry me. She said yes, and we were married about six months later.

We came very close to having to cancel the wedding at the last minute. I found out Barbara's divorce from her second husband had not been finalized. We hired an attorney who located him and got him to immediately agree to the divorce. That was only two days before the wedding.

Her mother, brother, and sister came with their children. My parents and Marie attended. I was flying high on this new beginning. My life was being totally turned around.

We both said, "I do" at the appropriate time, and we led everyone to a nearby restaurant where we celebrated over lunch.

Two days later we were on our way to the Dominican Republic where we celebrated our honeymoon at a romantic resort. It was one of the best weeks of my life. The dream come true just kept getting better and better. We relaxed on the beach, played in the pool where there was a swim-up bar, and held hands nearly all the time. One vivid memory I still have is slow dancing with Barbara in the moonlight on the concourse to the faint music of a distant saxophone. I certainly wasn't alone anymore.

As soon as we returned from the wonderful time in the Dominican Republic, we had to deal with both personal and business-related financial problems. Barbara had a huge stack of unpaid bills, and debt collectors called all of the time. Some checks she used to pay her bills were returned for insufficient funds. I felt I had no choice but to help her with her rather substantial debt.

Meanwhile Barbara and her business partner didn't realize that a large percentage of new businesses fail. They didn't realize it usually took at least a year or more for even a successful business to start making a profit. They believed the franchise executive who gave them the impression they could start making a profit soon after they opened.

Since Barbara was staffing the women's exercise studio, she planned to take money from the receipts so she could survive. One problem was there wasn't enough money left over after they paid for the rent and some franchise fees.

Another issue was that Barbara's partner expected Barbara to put what she took out of the business back in once they got the exercise studio turning a nice profit.

It seemed to me that Barbara was really being taken advantage of. She was expected to work for free even though she had invested just as much as her partner.

I explained this to Barbara. She got very upset and went to her mother for advice. Her mom had her accountant go over the numbers, and he told her that there wouldn't be enough money to support Barbara for quite some time even if the business was successful.

He also told her he thought they would need to invest more money before they could achieve even a chance of solvency. They would have to develop a marketing plan, including some local advertising, so that they could get enough new members to make a difference. He told them they would be better off cutting their losses and shutting down the new women's exercise club. Even with the additional investment there was no guarantee of future profitability. There were two successful Curves franchises in the general area that they were competing with.

We put a notice on the door stating it was closed until further notice. Barbara's partner sold the equipment back to the franchise company for a fraction of what they paid for it.

So Barbara lost both her mother's investment and her dream of running a successful business. She also lost her best friend from high school. This was not a great way to start a marriage. Neither Barbara nor I were working then. I had to start cashing in my investments right away to help pay $4,000 to $5,000 of Barb's previous debts. She also owed thousands for back property taxes, but I wouldn't discover that for at least another year.

Chapter 16

A few months after our honeymoon we invited Marie and all of Barbara's family to join us for our first Christmas together. Barbara wanted to have her entire family see how happy she was since I joined her and her girls. The dinner seemed to be a success. Everyone seemed to be having a good time. There was lots of catching up on family news. Barbara's brother Patrick kept going outside every fifteen or twenty minutes to drink more than he wanted his family to see. Patrick was having serious problems in his marriage. Apparently Patrick had sex with his wife the night before. It was the first time in a long time, and Patrick pulled me aside to tell me about it. He had a huge smile. Maybe she would stick with him after all. Barbara's brother was the first person to leave the gathering. He left a pile of empty beer cans on our front lawn.

About half of our guests had left when the phone rang. It was Patrick's daughter with horrible news. She had arrived at her home to find her father asleep on the living room couch. She tried to wake him, but he wouldn't move. He was dead. It was a freak accident. Patrick passed out from drinking too much and he choked to death on his own vomit. Our first Christmas together was a terrible time especially for Barbara and her mother. Their sadness and mourning was contagious.

My illness took advantage of the terrible situation and kept me in a depression at holiday time that should have been really happy for the newlyweds. I even had some hallucinations and delusional thinking. I didn't know it at the time but it turned out Barbara suffered from a personality disorder and was dealing with her own symptoms.

A few months after Patrick died, Barbara's mother was admitted to the hospital with a broken hip. She fell down trying to board a downtown train she took to get to her office every day. She managed to drag herself off the train after it arrived downtown.

She tried to do her job, but the pain was just too severe. She went to a hospital emergency room and was admitted. We visited her there, and she seemed like she was recovering just fine. I took a walk around the hospital so Barbara could have some private time with her mom.

During a routine check-up before her discharge a doctor found advanced stage cancer in Barbara's mom. She died of that cancer in that same hospital about a month after it was discovered.

Barbara was totally devastated. She recently lost her dream of owning her own business and her best friend. She had two failed marriages. Her brother and her mother were the relatives she felt closest to. Over the years she had confided in them with her personal issues. Now they were both dead.

After these tragic losses, Barbara was never quite the same. I hoped that my experience with profound loss could somehow help me to help her. It may have in a very limited way because I understood how she was feeling, but I soon discovered that nothing I could do or say could make a difference in her thoughts and behavior.

Despite our wonderful romance and terrific honeymoon, our marriage became rather toxic. I wanted to continue the feelings we had during our honeymoon. I wanted us to be even closer than we were. Barbara felt much more comfortable with considerably more distance between us. She felt an almost desperate need to leave the house without me and do things by herself. Sometimes when this happened I would believe she was seeing someone else. So we were constantly pulling and pushing each other in and out of our lives together.

At first I blamed Barbara's desperate need to be without me as the sole problem of the marriage. Now I know it wasn't all Barbara's fault. We both were making it difficult for our marriage to bring us mutual happiness. It was like we pulled some switch that turned our marriage on its head.

After we lived together for about eight months, her deceased brother's first wife called to invite Barbara to join her and her boyfriend that evening at an indoor swimming pool. I was definitely not invited. The boyfriend was bringing one of his friends too, so there would be two couples at the pool.

One would be Barbara and the man she didn't know. I thought this was totally inappropriate for a married woman and told her so. We got into quite a fight over it, but she went anyway.

After she left, the pain of the lonely night woke up my inert suicidal madness. After the girls went to bed, I waited and waited for Barbara to come home.

I had a lump in my throat and pain in my stomach. I had tears in my eyes. I was paralyzed by inner pain. Hours went by. There was no way she could still be at the pool. I could only imagine what was keeping her out this late. Was she in the stranger's arms? Was she starting an affair?

The phone rang about 11 p.m. It was her brother's first wife. She told me Barbara had been drinking and she was just too tired to drive home.

Would I mind if she stayed the night at her house and drove home in the morning? She made it sound so innocent. Suicidal madness was exploding in my brain. I told her if Barbara didn't get home until the morning she wouldn't find me here. I would be long gone. I would leave her for certain.

Barbara got on the phone, and I told her I would kill myself if she didn't come straight home. I meant it. I assumed she wanted to spend all night long with another man. I just couldn't bear the inner pain of her being with another man for the entire night.

This would have caused any spouse terrible internal suffering. In my case my madness made the pain so severe, all I wanted to do was end it by ending my life. Barbara knew about my suicidal history, and she walked in the front door about an hour later. I didn't know whether to hug her or hit her.

I sat on the front porch by myself painfully watching the sun rise not knowing what the rest of the day would bring. Barbara's former sister-in-law showed up later that morning. I guess she wanted to check for herself to make sure Barbara was okay. After talking with Barbara for a while, she came out on the porch to visit with me. I was ashamed of my suicidal behavior, and I was speechless in her company. I didn't want to scream at her so I was silent.

Even though I was so upset I could barely speak, I wanted to hold Barbara and love her. She claimed nothing happened. At first I had a very hard time believing her, but I ended up hoping she was right.

Regardless of her complaints, I really wanted to make her happy. I bought very expensive tickets for popular shows. We saw Jerry Seinfeld's one-man show. I paid more than $1300 for tickets for Elton John and considerably more than that for good tickets to see the Rolling Stones.

This was her second Rolling Stones concert. She made a big deal about her first concert. The seats were much closer and better than the tickets I bought for us.

I did everything I could think of to restore our closeness, but the more I spent, the further she pushed herself away from me. She accused me of "lording over her" with my money.

After we were married about two years, Barbara announced one day that she would be going away for three days over the weekend to attend a Catholic retreat.

I was surprised. Even though we went to Sunday mass once in a while, she wasn't particularly religious. She wouldn't tell me much about it other than she just had to attend it for her spiritual growth. At the time I still didn't understand her need to do things all by herself. I didn't know where it was, what its theme was, or why she was so intent on going there alone. She said she would be gone for three days and two nights.

Where would she be staying on those nights? Was this going to be another swimming pool incident, only one that lasted for three days instead of one night?

I remembered how easy it seemed to her when she had that long affair while she was married to her first husband. I wondered how her first husband tolerated her travels, her one-person vacations and her busy mysterious days. She rationalized her behavior by saying her first husband avoided her on weekends when he was home from work.

He would set up shop in the garage where he and his friends would watch football and drink beer. She said he was controlling, manipulative, and distant. She was so tired of not having her emotional needs cared for.

Although I never drank beer in the garage with my buddies, I received almost the same type of complaints she continually had about her first husband.

I was controlling. I often tried to manipulate her. I was selfish. I didn't pay enough attention to her and her emotional needs.

Her strong need not to be with me, to reject my loving feelings by leaving me alone while she went off by herself or to meet others I didn't know—all this sometimes triggered my suicidal thoughts and behavior. A couple of times a man called asking for Barbara when she wasn't home. He didn't identify himself or leave a message. I assumed the worst. Years later a friend told me she saw Barbara with another man attending group meetings at a local church.

Now I can see how she thought my suicidal behavior was an effort to manipulate her, but it was really caused by my manic depression triggered by her efforts to push me away. If I wasn't mentally ill, I would not have become suicidal.

Normal people did not seriously flirt with suicide like I did.

In sessions with Dr. Francis I realized that my relationship with Barbara was a lot like my relationship with Maura in its final years. I totally depended on them for any feelings of self-worth. I had nothing of my own to make me feel good about myself. Whether I felt good or bad depended solely on the immediate state of my relationships.

Neither of us was able to find work for a long time. I paid for everything by cashing in my investments. I also borrowed $40,000 in my name by obtaining a second mortgage for her house. And we maxed out my Mastercard for about $30,000. I had to replace the sump pump and pay around $17,000 for a new sewer line in the back yard. The house really needed painting. It was an eyesore of peeling paint. The girls must have been ashamed of it when their friends came over. So I paid to have it painted.

Her stove, dishwasher, and refrigerator needed to be replaced so I bought new ones. When we married I discovered she had about $5,000 of bills that needed to be paid. These expenditures were in addition to the thousands we spent each month on the mortgage, groceries, clothes, and other basic living expenses. She was getting child support from the girls' father. I was still receiving disability benefits from Social Security and the last few payments from an annuity. Every few months I would have to ask Harry to cash in thousands of dollars from my investments. He always tried to talk me out of it, but I had no other choice. I was the husband and stepfather. I was supposed to pay for the needs of my new family.

Barbara found employment at the local Walgreens. It didn't pay a lot, but it was enough to take care of our primary mortgage. So she paid for the mortgage, and I paid for everything else. After several months of this arrangement a man came to our front door and gave us a foreclosure notice.

It said we missed four consecutive mortgage payments. The payments were supposed to be taken from Barbara's checking account. They weren't because Barbara didn't call each month to approve the payments as was the bank's policy.

Barbara's excuse was she didn't know that they didn't take the mortgage payments from her account. Who doesn't look at their checking account balance for several months at a time?

We couldn't lose the house. I called the bank and pleaded with them to get us out of foreclosure. I told them the missed payments came from a misunderstanding. Nothing I said mattered to them. To get us out of foreclosure I had to pay around $15,000 plus about $2,500 a month for six months. Finally, I discovered Barbara owed around $5,000 in back property taxes I had to pay.

Barbara was having difficulty with her job at Walgreens. They told her she should have friendly chats with customers. She loved her conversations with customers, but it kept her from completing other tasks such as stocking the empty shelves. She complained about how her boss treated her all the time. He wanted her to stock shelves and visit with customers. She couldn't do both, she said. He should make up his mind about what he really wanted her to do.

After working there for about a year, she came home early one day and told me she couldn't take the way her boss treated her anymore so she quit. I always thought she was probably fired, but I didn't mention that to her.

We both continued looking for work. It had been a long time since I inhabited the upper ranks of corporate America.

I applied at local stores to no avail. After reading my resume they must have thought I was overqualified. I went for an interview with Holy Family Church. It was a progressive Catholic church looking for someone to work part-time and put together a newsletter to bring public attention to their many community programs. For example, they had a program that brought divorced single people together in hopes that they would find a match. I never heard back.

I wrote the new CEO of Sears. He had been the senior vice president of finance for Kraft when I worked there. The VP of Sears in charge of public relations called me. He told me his CEO asked him to call. He told me I had terrific experience in my profession, but he didn't have any openings for me.

Richard Edelman, the CEO of the Edelman Public Relations Agency headquartered in New York City, set me up for interviews at his Chicago office. He wanted to help me. I had worked with his agency in both New York and Chicago.

I went on the interviews thinking this was a terrific opportunity for me to get back into my profession. After all, when the CEO recommends you, it is almost automatic that you get hired. I must have really failed at these interviews, and they obviously knew about my bipolar illness. When it was all said and done, I received good wishes and some encouragement for my future but no job offer.

The *Chicago Tribune* editor who handled my column on Mark's death introduced me to the reporter who wrote mental health stories. She gave me practical advice on how to sell freelance writing.

Again, they really wished me well. I never tried freelance writing. It seemed like too much work for even the possibility of selling an article to a publication.

Every employment possibility started with hope and ended up in rejections that fueled my manic-depressive sadness.

A friend of mine who still worked in the Philip Morris corporate communications department hired me to write two different speeches for top executives.

They paid $1,000 a speech. I used the money to help get our house out of foreclosure. The speech assignment was a one-time deal, a friend helping a friend. The company had professional speechwriters it had been using for many years.

I eventually got a part-time job as a reporter for *The Daily Herald*, a large suburban Chicago daily newspaper. One of the editors asked me to attend various evening meetings of local elected government officials from suburban cities.

These meetings lasted for a few hours. I had to determine what news was coming from the gatherings of small-town officials. The arrival of new stores or housing developments or office buildings was important news for *Herald* readers. I did one series that ended up on the front page on how coyotes were terrorizing suburban communities. Several small dogs had been attacked by gangs of coyotes.

The job paid only $40 a story. That included the hours spent at the meetings and the time spent writing the stories the next morning. The pay was terrible, but the work got my name in the paper, "by Tom Ricke." I never got tired of that.

I averaged six meetings a month. Sometimes there would be two stories from a meeting. It never took me more than thirty minutes to write a story. I could write newspaper stories in my sleep.

This all was before I had GPS. I got easily confused and had a hard time finding the buildings where evening municipal meetings were held. I had a lot of difficulty navigating in the dark. So I found the buildings in the afternoon when I wrote down the directions for that evening.

I earned a lot more than money while I worked for the *Daily Herald*. My self-esteem came out of hiding, and slowly and surely made every aspect of my life better.

Dr. Francis told me that working at the *Daily Herald* turned my life around. She said I was better than I had been for the previous four years. I was not troubled so much by Barbara's need to go out by herself. I liked myself much better.

One day the phone calls asking me to cover the meetings just stopped. I called my editor and he didn't return my calls. He had been promoted to business editor and his replacement at the news desk had his own stringer to cover the evening meetings.

Meanwhile Barbara had discovered a company that was interviewing for outside sales reps. We were driving somewhere when I told her I wanted to go with her and have my own interview. Maybe they would hire both of us.

She froze. She felt the immediate need to get away from me and be alone. As I was slowing down before a traffic light, she opened her door and jumped out of the car and ran away.

I parked the car near the intersection and looked everywhere for her. I looked in an auto repair shop, a restaurant, a convenience store, and a gas station. I looked at these nearby places again. She wasn't there the second time either. I didn't know what to do so I called the police. They showed up a few minutes later. I had called

Barbara's cell several times since she jumped out of the car, and she didn't answer. I tried again in front of the police and she answered it.

She was standing in front of a Barnes and Noble book store about a mile away. The police told her to stay there and sent a car to pick her up.

When she arrived police asked her if I had been violent with her. She said I wasn't, and then the police tried to make light of our situation. They told us that jumping out of cars was more common than you would think. They called them "jumpers."

We drove home as if nothing had happened. I thought about teasing her by calling her "jumper," but I didn't do it. We had enough drama for one day.

Chapter 17

I continued to have lunch with Harry every few weeks. When I saw him I would ask for statements on what I had left with the Fidelity investments. He would lecture me for cashing in some of them to meet my expenses but always told me the statements were coming. Nearly two years passed by. I never saw a statement.

I thought of Harry as a good friend, and I didn't have many friends. I was shy about asking him for the documentation. I would wait until lunch was over before I brought it up. I didn't want to hurt our friendship. I just couldn't believe he would cheat me so I didn't make a big deal about not having statements from Fidelity. He must have a good reason for not giving them to me. Maybe he put my funds together with some of his investments or with another person's accounts.

Fidelity is a very reputable company. It must have provided statements about the investments, but I had no idea who received them. It wasn't me. It occurred to me that if there continued to be a big problem with Harry handling my money, it could end up being his word against mine. Who would be believed? The financial advisor or his mentally ill client?

I knew I had to do something about Harry and my money. I finally went to an attorney I had used once before. She said she would write a stern letter to Harry asking for my money back. Harry called and screamed at me over the phone when he received the letter. We were friends. How could I turn on him like this?

When I told my family about my situation with Harry, they told me he was taking advantage of me due to my mental illness. I still had not seen any statements from Fidelity. I had no idea of what he had done with my money.

In the end he wrote me a check for what I gave him from cashing in the annuities minus the substantial funds I had to withdraw to get us out of foreclosure and pay for home maintenance and all the other expenses with Barbara.

After my withdrawals I had less than half of what I started with. I didn't get a dime for investment returns on what was left, not even the meager interest it would have earned in a bank's saving account. All I got back was what was left of the principal investment, but it could have been much worse if he had kept all of my money.

In spite of all this I tried to remain friends with Harry. I felt I couldn't afford to lose a friend. I thought he was a good man. He took me shopping for furniture when I really needed it. He said he would be there for me whenever I needed or wanted his company.

I didn't realize it at the time, but he needed my friendship as much as I needed his. We resumed our casual lunches and never again spoke about the finances.

Meanwhile Barbara and I tried to lead a normal life— husband, wife and two children. We would succeed for a while, but what I now realize were symptoms of my manic depression and her personality disorder would make it very difficult for us to get along at times.

She was up and down, mean and nice and mean again. Looking back, I now see that money issues were a much bigger factor in her treatment of me than I realized at the time. When she was in financial need she would be affectionate and caring. She would cook a nice dinner instead of our usual diet of take-out food. We would make love. I would feel like my dreams of a wonderful marriage were coming true.

Then after I paid whatever debt or bill was looming at the time, she turned into the mean and cruel Barbara. She was not the least bit grateful for my financial assistance. She seemed to be punishing me for helping her. She must have been ashamed of her continuing fiscal crisis, ashamed and angry that she needed my help in the first place.

We went to three different marriage counselors looking for the assistance that could bring us back together is a healthy, mutually satisfying marriage.

I tried my best to remain optimistic no matter how negative Barbara became. I wanted to stay married. I would have done anything to realize the potential I believed we had for being truly happy together. She said she did too. We had some good moments and good times but never for very long.

During the sessions she was the victim of my harsh and cruel and insensitive treatment. I was to blame for all the trouble in her life. She had no problem spending the whole hour complaining about me. However, when the counselor turned the tables and began to focus on her behavior and attitude, Barbara would shut down and refuse to cooperate any longer. When the last of three marriage counselors started to bring our attention to Barbara's stark negativity, she got up, left the room, and drove away. The counselor told me it was too bad she was so scared. He felt we had enough love and appreciation to make the marriage work. That was our last session with marriage counseling.

We went for days walking on eggshells afraid to speak to each other and risk more emotional scenes. Sometimes when she was really upset she would take off her wedding rings. She left more frequently, not telling me where she was going and when she would be back home.

One time when Marie was visiting, Barbara stayed in the bathroom for more than an hour waiting for Marie to leave before she came out. I never did understand what that was all about.

We tried not to fight in front of the girls, but we still had our confrontations. Sometimes we would go into our bedroom and shut the door while we argued in whispers.

Our disagreements seemed to be based on the difference in our emotional needs. I wanted us to be closer, and she was much more comfortable with us further apart.

Things became less heated after I followed Dr. Francis's advice and wrote down my feelings instead of shouting about them, but sometimes it was very hard not to be really upset.

She went out to lunch with a former boss and didn't get home until 7 p.m. Another time I was talking to Marie, and Maura came on the line to say hello. Barbara listened while I talked with Maura. I don't remember what I said, but it may have been something inappropriate. I didn't talk with Maura very often, but when I did, I wanted her to know I still cared for her. Barbara was so upset with whatever I said, she took off her wedding rings and stormed out of the house.

We were together for less than three years before it got so bad she wanted us to break up. Although she talked about a divorce once in a while she never came out and asked me to leave. When she was with friends and relatives, she was the life of the party. She had a great sense of humor. When she was with me she was a different person altogether. I had become the enemy. I was the reason for every big problem she had.

We weren't a couple anymore, just a man and woman living in the same house. It broke my heart.

Suicide began to seduce me. I was working on a long letter about my hurt feelings that I was going to give to Barbara. It was easy to turn it into a suicide note. The pain from Barbara's rejections and hurtful language was crippling my ability to function normally. I wanted immediate relief, and I really wanted her to know just how much she was hurting me.

Marriages break up all of the time, but people don't kill themselves over it. I was the exception. I finally stepped over the line on Halloween.

Children from our section of the neighborhood skipped from house to house collecting their candy. A group of parents walked behind them on the street. A side effect of one of my medications made me walk slowly. No matter how hard I tried to catch up, Barbara would not walk with me.

She walked with neighbors ahead of me. It was the second Halloween in a row that I ended up walking all alone in the back of the crowd. Every painful step I took seemed to move me closer to the end. After about an hour I left the group and walked back to our house where I put the final touches on my suicide note.

I was still working on it when Barbara and her younger daughter came home. Her older daughter was still out with some of her friends.

I decided to end my life in a nearby Holiday Inn. I wanted to protect the girls and not have them discover my body. I packed up all of my drugs into a large plastic bag. I gave the letter to Barbara on my way out the door. Another failed marriage. Another dose of unbearable inner pain. Another life lost, again.

When I checked into the hotel, I had no luggage, just the big bag of pills. The clerk who gave me keys to a room didn't make a comment. As the old joke goes, I was checking into the "no-tell motel."

After I closed the door and walked into my room, I had some decisions to make. The first was choosing which pills to take.

I had read somewhere that lithium was very toxic and dangerous. I had a recently refilled prescription of lithium. So I opened the bottle and began to wash the pills down my throat two to three at a time.

I stopped after two or three handfuls to make a couple of phone calls. I left a goodbye message for Dr. Francis.

One of Dr. Easton's partners who was covering for him that night answered my call. After I gave him the goodbye message meant for Dr. Easton he tried the best he could to talk me out of it. I hung up before he finished his plea.

Then I called Barbara to give her a proper goodbye. I told her my passing wasn't her fault. My manic depression was ruling the night.

Barbara had called the police so she gave the phone to a sheriff's deputy who had responded to her call. He tried to talk me into coming home. He gave the phone back to Barbara when he realized nothing he could say to me was going to stop me.

I kept thinking about what was going to happen to my car which I left in the parking lot.

So I made the mistake of telling Barbara where she could find the car the following morning.

I went back to taking the pills. After a few more handfuls the phone rang.

It was Dr. Easton returning my earlier call. His partner must have tracked him down and told him to call me.

He begged me to call the police. Just then there was someone knocking at the door. Two policemen were standing in the hallway outside my room.

Barbara must have told them where I was since she knew where my car was parked. When I refused to answer the door, they told me that they would break the door down if I wouldn't let them in.

There was an ambulance waiting for me near the front door of the hotel.

They took me to the emergency room at Northwestern Community Hospital.

I didn't know it at the time, but Dr. Easton stayed on the phone for a long time as the ER doctors tried to cleanse the lithium from my blood.

At first the doctors told me to take bites of a black brick that seemed to be made of charcoal. I argued with them. I didn't want to be saved.

They told me if I didn't eat some of the black brick they would forcefully pump my stomach. As soon as I took a couple of bites my insides exploded.

There was a toilet out in the open with absolutely no privacy. I had to empty my bowels there and vomited the contents of my stomach while I was sure everyone was staring at me.

The pooping and vomiting must not have totally removed the toxic lithium from my system. Soon after I returned from the wide open toilet they forced a tube into my nose and down to my stomach. As they pumped my stomach, I could see the liquid contents move through the tube. I was not happy that they seemed to be saving me.

After they received the results of how much lithium was still in my blood they sat me down next to a dialysis machine and stuck a very large needle in my neck. The treatment worked and I was shipped off to the thirteenth floor of Rush University Medical Center, the psychiatric ward I used to live in.

A few days after my admission I called Barbara and asked her to come downtown to visit me. It was a Sunday afternoon and the girls were with their father. Much to my surprise she drove for more than an hour to see me. I was so happy to see her, so happy she cared enough to visit me I thought that everything would be much better when I got back home.

I switched from suicidal depression to an affectionate mania.

I had been diagnosed as suffering from rapid cycling manic depression. This cycling was certainly rapid.

I started a campaign to get home as soon as possible. They let me out in a few more days. When Dr. Easton and the psychiatrists in his practice reviewed my case, they decided they should have kept me in the hospital for at least another week.

Barbara did not welcome me home. She didn't really want to see me.

I was so disappointed. I went out and bought a bottle of wine which I hid in the upstairs study. It took me three days of self-medicating to finish the bottle.

I felt some comfort from the first alcohol I had consumed in a very long time, but I defied the traditional AA thinking that a person who was once an alcoholic can never drink safely again. I did not get drunk or tipsy.

I continued drinking moderately from then until now without ever getting drunk. I know my story is rather unique. I would not recommend drinking to anyone with a drinking problem, but for some reason it was okay for me.

Dr. Francis was astonished that I could drink safely after decades of Antabuse-reinforced sobriety. Dr. Easton said that there was a recent study that determined some problem drinkers could drink again when they got older.

I think I was self-medicating with liquor when I abused it, and I abused it all of the time when I was drinking. Now that I am being medicated with several prescriptions, perhaps I don't need to self-medicate so much. Whatever the reason, I can take it or leave now. The most I ever have is two drinks. After that I don't want any more.

Over the next few months it became clear to me that I would have to leave my new family so that Barbara could get the divorce she said she wanted. I started to get ready for the move. I bought a few items I would really need: a coffee pot, a phone, a bed, mattress, and bed clothes. I put a down payment on an apartment in the same huge complex I lived in before I married Barbara, but I didn't move in right away.

I made myself go through the motions of the breakup she wanted. As usual she was off and on about us, but much more off than on.

When things were better, I would think about saving money by getting rid of the empty apartment I was renting, but I kept it.

Despite a few expressions of mutual affection and some hope for a future together, I knew deep down that our days were numbered. Every day I took steps leading to my leaving for good.

After going through at least two-thirds of the investments I had saved for my retirement including the $30,000 spent to get her out of foreclosure, after all of her blaming me for the problems in her life, after all those hurtful words and actions, I would have stayed if she asked me to.

Until the moving van showed up I was hoping she would change her mind.

I stopped my monthly payments on the second mortgage when I moved out. Barbara had a new job and she agreed to take over those payments, but she never did. The bank came after me for years. My credit was ruined.

I still had to pay off $35,000 on the Mastercard account we shared. In spite of all this I still wanted to stay with Barbara even though I knew she would continue to deplete what was left of my retirement savings.

She never had any money to speak of. Her pay at the new job was based on sales commissions she would earn if and when her company signed contracts with potential customers she identified from initial phone calls. She couldn't pay what she didn't have.

I still wanted her to find secure happiness in her life even if it wouldn't be with me. I told myself it wasn't her fault that she had such a horrible childhood. It was no more her fault that she had a personality disorder than it was my fault I was bipolar.

I told myself she was a good person trapped in a life without luck and without the ability to sustain the loving relationship she said she wanted.

Even though I moved out, I still hoped somehow that we could get back together for a second chance.

From time to time we had to talk on the phone about some of the unresolved issues of our breakup. For example, all of her older daughter's music was on my computer and she needed to come over and get it. I wasn't able to bring everything when I moved, so Barbara offered to put my things in boxes for me.

At first the conversations we had after I left were her usual one-sided criticisms of me. I was just no good and the cause of all of her problems.

After several months Barbara calmed down, and we were able to be more civilized and concerned for whatever might have been left of the relationship. Suddenly she was very nice and seemed interested in seeing me in person. I was terribly lonely. I was so very sad. As long as she was civil to me, I dared to hope for a successful second chance.

My longing to be with Barbara again became stronger. I thought she must have felt the same way. We started back with a Friday night date. I took her out for dinner then we went to the casino in Elgin. On the way from the parking lot to the casino I took her hand, and she squeezed mine.

The next time we went out we went to the movies. I brought her flowers and we made love in my apartment at the end of the evening and again on the following day. We continued this dating for months. Each time I brought flowers. Each time we made love.

I told myself not to get too serious about what was turning out to be an affair with my own wife, but I couldn't help thinking we were heading back together permanently.

She must have been thinking that too. She began cooking Sunday dinners for me and the girls. It turns out they were also hoping that I would move back in.

My family cautioned me about seeing Barbara again. They worried that all she really wanted from me was what was left of my retirement savings. Even with her child support and money earned on the new job, she didn't have enough money to pay her bills. She wasn't extravagant. She didn't spend a lot of money on herself. At least that's what I told myself when she asked to borrow another $1,200.

She asked for the "loan" she needed as a down payment on a mortgage she had applied for. This new mortgage would give her a monthly payment that would be considerably lower than a separate first and second mortgage. She promised to pay me back when she received the proceeds from the mortgage.

For her it was more comfortable to date the way we were than to live together again. We could still fulfill our mutual passion without the closeness that comes from sleeping in the same bed every night. Act two was terrific for both of us, until it wasn't.

At first Marie really liked Barbara. She was happy I had met her. But, over time, she began to distrust Barbara. Sometimes when I talked to Marie on the phone, she could tell I was very upset with the way Barbara was treating me.

She could tell I was depressed. Even though I wouldn't talk about it with her, she feared I was suicidal. She would cry sometimes after we hung up. She began to hate Barbara for the way she treated me. She saw a woman taking financial advantage of her mentally ill father.

I did share my financial concerns with Marie and my parents.

They both warned me not to trust Barbara with more money.

Since she considered the $1,200 a loan she would repay I ignored their warnings.

It turned out that they were right. She never got the mortgage. She spent the money on a car and never paid me back, and she didn't even make one payment on the second mortgage.

It had become our Ricke family tradition that Marie would spend Christmas with her mother and Thanksgiving with me. When I lived alone Marie would come to my apartment and we would cook a traditional Thanksgiving dinner.

On this particular Thanksgiving Barbara and I were dating again, and I was really in a bind. Marie would hate it if Barbara was with us on our special day. Barbara could be all alone if I didn't ask her to join us. When we talked about Thanksgiving in general Barbara mentioned that she already had plans. I thought that would solve my Thanksgiving problem, but it didn't.

On the weekend before Thanksgiving Barbara told me that someone in her family had asked her why she wasn't spending the holiday with her husband instead of with her girls' grandparents. After all, they told her, since you are getting back together you should be with your husband on this special day. She had tears in her eyes when she told me this.

The only thing I could think of was to split the holiday in two. I would have my Thanksgiving meal with Marie in the early afternoon. Then I would spend the late afternoon and evening with Barbara.

Although Barbara was very upset with the situation, she told me again not to worry because she had other plans. I don't know for sure, but now I think she could have been all alone on that Thanksgiving.

The next time we got together it was for a movie and dinner. She told me she wouldn't have time for our weekly session in my apartment. She would have to leave right after dinner because her daughter was out on a date, and Barbara wanted to be home when her daughter came home.

As soon as the movie was over Barbara stood up and bolted out of the theatre leaving me trying to keep up with her. One of her daughter's friends was working as a ticket taker in that theatre. He saw Barbara fly to the doors with me in hot pursuit.

"I thought you two were getting back together," he said as I passed him.

"I thought so too," I replied.

Barbara didn't stay for dinner. She ran to her car and sped away leaving me standing alone in the parking lot. That turned out to be the end of our second (and last) act. The next time I saw her was in court.

Chapter 18

After Barbara and I split up for good I felt more sad than ever. Most of the work I did on my evening job at Good Shepherd happened after 5 p.m. when the majority of employees went home. I often spent my late hours doing mindless paperwork in an office all by myself.

Occasionally I would have a conversation with a volunteer that was more than a hello or goodbye or comments about the weather. When I would take a teen volunteer to his or her workstation on patient floors, I would speak to nurses as I introduced the new volunteer for the unit.

During this time I learned you could be quite lonely even if you were surrounded by people. Hundreds of doctors, nurses, and administrators cared for the patients over three shifts. As superficial as my short conversations with others in the hospital were, they were better than the painful quiet of being alone in my apartment where a television was my only companion.

The job did get me out of the house five days a week. It did give me the opportunity to communicate with others, and it did provide good health insurance.

Some of the volunteer positions were critical, and if the volunteer for that specific job didn't show up sometimes I would have to fill in.

It took two volunteers to staff what we called the front desk of the hospital, where the volunteers greeted guests and handed out visitor passes. From time to time I would have to work there. I liked it because it kept me busy and it gave me the opportunity to get to know the volunteer I was working with as we would chat throughout the evening.

I had several front desk evenings when I shared the desk duties with a young woman named Beth. We talked a lot, and during one of our conversations about what I needed to feel less lonely in my life, I mentioned that I missed having a dog. Maura and I always had a dog while we were raising our family.

Beth invited me to a couple of parties at her house where she had a group of relatives and friends. I was grateful for her thoughtfulness, but I felt slow and awkward and out of place. Everyone there knew one another, and all the guests were busy talking to one another. Some played board games or card games. I stood alone not sure of what I should do or say next.

Beth rescued me a couple of times by introducing me to people talking in groups. She worked in a chiropractor's office, and several of her co-workers were there. They were talking about back surgery and how dangerous it was compared to chiropractors' treatments.

At that time I just had back surgery, but I chose not to argue with them about the necessity for my operation. So I just stood there feeling stupid.

A few weeks later Beth and her teenage son surprised me by coming to my apartment. I had no idea how she got my address. She told me to put on my jacket, that we were going to get a dog.

The first two shelters we visited had only pit bulls that had bitten people and were waiting to be put down. They looked cute, but I didn't want to take a chance on any of them. We had one stop left. Beth wanted us to check out a shelter in Lincolnshire called Orphans of the Storm. The shelter did not have any of its dogs put down, and it had more than fifty dogs waiting to be rescued.

As soon as we walked in a teenage girl walked up to us and asked us if we were there to adopt a dog. I hardly had time to answer her before she grabbed my arm and led me to a cute little dog in a nearby cage. She said, "His name is Lucky, and he is adorable. He is so affectionate he will sit on your lap while you watch TV."

She put a leash on him and invited me to take him for a short walk in back of their property. The sixteen-pound rat terrier was seducing me. When we got back to the main building, I sat down and Lucky jumped in my lap and licked my hand. I knew I had found my dog. They said he was four years old. He hadn't been fixed, and they would not release him until he was neutered.

We arranged to have him fixed at a local animal hospital. I would be able to pick him up the next day. I took him home ten years ago, and he has been with me ever since.

Even though I had my part-time job at Good Shepherd Hospital, during those years I still had some lonely and depressing times. I would get home around 8:30 p.m. every weekday night. Everything was dark and quiet and sad. There was no one to talk to. No one to share smiles or frowns. No one to go through the daily motions of life with. You can only watch so much television.

I was all alone one Christmas. It was late in the evening. I was hungry. I hadn't eaten all day and there was nothing good to eat in the fridge. I would have to go out to get something. Everyplace I could think of was closed.

After more than thirty minutes I drove by a McDonald's. I couldn't see anyone inside, but the lights were on, and it seemed to be open. I parked the car and walked in.

There was one man in the store. He was standing back in the kitchen, and he seemed surprised that he had a customer so late on Christmas day.

I ordered a Big Mac, fries, and a Diet Coke. When I reached into my back pocket to get my wallet, it wasn't there. I had left it at home.

I apologized and turned to leave when the man called me back.

He must have felt really sorry for me because he gave me my order for free. I thanked him and left with the food, but I felt so terrible. All alone on Christmas. All alone in a McDonald's without my wallet. So very far from the wonderful Christmases with Maura, Mark, and Marie. I felt I was trapped in a black tar of despair. I shuffled out of the store and drove home. I ate my dinner and drove back to the McDonald's to pay for it.

That Christmas night was a very sad time for me. I drove home and tried playing with Lucky, but I couldn't. It just hurt too much. I sat and stared at the television. Every breath hurt. Every moment hurt. Living itself was all pain. The good news was I didn't attempt another suicide. I eventually fell asleep and woke up to another day of sorrow. I was used to it and I got through the day by just putting one foot in front of the other taking slow, purposeful steps through the sad moments. I was shuffling through a pile of dark Jell-O.

Marie and Jim met at a wedding in Texas where they both missed their return flights because they were lost in each other's conversations. Jim lived and worked in Washington, DC. They talked on the phone nearly every day, and they took turns visiting each other.

Every few weeks I would pick Marie up from the airport after she returned from a visit with Jim.

He eventually moved to Chicago so he and Marie could see each other all the time. Marie had a good job as a speech therapist. Jim had worked as a consultant for a government agency.

He did very well in Washington, but when he looked hard for a job in the Chicago area, he was unable to find one. After nearly a year Marie and Jim moved to Washington where they lived together in a small apartment near the airport.

There is a great need for speech therapists just about everywhere.

Marie had a job offer from a DC clinic where she would be working with small children. She called it her dream job. Jim was able to get a good job with a large national consulting firm where he worked with a government agency. They were very happy together.

One night when I was feeling pretty good, Jim called me. He asked for my permission to marry Marie. Of course I said yes but wondered what would have happened if I had not approved.

The outdoor wedding took place on a small lake near Richmond, Virginia. I flew there and rented a car. My job, of course, was to walk Marie down the aisle and bring her to Jim who was standing next to the preacher. I could feel every eye in the audience staring at Marie and me as we walked on the wet grass on our journey to the altar. They were kind stares from friends and relatives who were familiar with my intense struggle with mental illness. They knew I had been hospitalized many times. They were aware of my shock treatments and the fact that I took several medications each day. They were pleasantly surprised that I seemed to be doing quite well as I walked Marie down the aisle. That was one of the best moments of my life.

The other wedding festivities were not so good for me. I was alone and felt different and out of place. It seemed like everyone was a couple except me. Maura was there with her new husband Jerry. My sisters and brother were there with their spouses. Maura's sister Mary came from Ireland with her husband.

There was a dinner the night before and a reception after the wedding.

For decades Maura and I socialized with the relatives and friends who attended Marie's wedding. At Marie's reception Maura and her husband sat with my brother and sisters and their spouses. The more they talked and laughed the more I felt all alone.

Dancing with Marie was wonderful. Dancing with Maura was not so good. Holding her close as we moved around the dance floor reminded me of the intimacy we shared in our good years together. It made me sad.

After the bride and groom left and the reception was over Maura and Jerry drove me back to the hotel. I felt like a little boy in the backseat of his parents' car.

Chapter 19

I met Gloria in a neighborhood bar where I was having dinner after work. I was eating alone at the bar, and she walked over and sat down next to me. We became friends and had dinner together once or twice a week. We were not intimate. We never even kissed or held hands. We were just good friends, and I was comfortable with that.

After Gloria and I were seeing each other for about six months, I realized I had to do something about my back. I was suffering with severe back pain. I got some relief when I sat down or lay down, but not enough to go through the motions of daily life without a crippling, screaming pain.

The first doctor I saw about my back gave me shots that took away the pain. I was living from shot to shot. I didn't miss any work. I hoped I would be able to live without the pain and not need shots in the future.

After more than a year the shots stopped working and the pain was worse than ever. The second doctor I saw was a back surgeon from Rush University Medical Center. He recommended what he called "minimally invasive" surgery.

I asked Gloria if she could come to the hospital with me so she could call my family after the surgery with what I hoped would be good news. At first she said she couldn't because she had planned a trip to Colorado that day. She needed to take care of some property she owned there.

Then she agreed to postpone her trip for a day so she could take me to the hospital very early in the morning and stay until the surgery was completed.

The surgeon told her the operation was a success, and she called my sister Peggy who shared the information with my parents and brother and sisters. Gloria left early the next morning.

I stayed as an inpatient for a couple of days. Since I had no one to pick me up I had to take a medical transport home. I had to walk up and down some steps to get to my apartment. I was alone and afraid I would fall. I made it home okay, but I was confined to the couch in my living room where I watched daytime TV. My only visitors were a nurse and a physical therapist. They each came every other day so I at least had a visitor for an hour or so every weekday.

After a week and a half I was able to go to the grocery store to replenish my supply of frozen dinners, lunchmeat, and fruit. After two weeks I was able to return to work. I used a cane to help me get around, but I only needed it for a month.

When Gloria returned from her trip we continued our routine of having dinner a couple of nights a week.

Not only was my back healing after the surgery, the symptoms of my manic depression were quieting down. I felt like I was getting a little better every month.

I was happy to have a normal job that had nothing to do with mental illness. When I worked at MHAI, I dealt with issues concerning people with mental illnesses during the day and my own symptoms at home during the evenings and weekends.

When I worked at Good Shepherd Hospital I didn't start until 4 p.m. so I had all day to deal with whatever minor symptoms may have been playing with me.

On days when I was sad I would watch movies on TV to keep my mind from heading down depression lane toward suicidal ideations.

On days I had a lot of energy, I would take Lucky for long walks, play with my email, and read suspenseful novels.

As time went by my symptoms continued to be milder and easier for me to keep hidden. After Barbara I was gun-shy and didn't look for romance for a couple of years.

Every once in a while I would go on the internet looking for a romantic relationship, but the results were always the same. When we met I may have been a little symptomatic, and when I told them I was bipolar they didn't want to see me again.

It was different with Marilee. I met her online at a seniors' dating service. After a couple of weeks of sending emails back and forth we talked on the phone. Before we could meet, my mother died at ninety-two, and I went to Sacramento to attend the services and spend some time with my father. Marilee's mother lived to be ninety-nine and died a few months earlier so we had something in common to talk about.

After I returned home Marilee and I agreed to meet and have dinner. She was early and waiting for me when I arrived. The front of the restaurant was filled with people without reservations who were waiting for a table.

Marilee came out of the crowd and tapped me on the shoulder. "I think you are looking for me," she said. She was wearing a black dress with tiny white polka-dots. Her smile was intoxicating. Her hair was red in a unique style that flattered her. She was very attractive. I thought about how my previous dates had ended up and wondered how long it would take for Marilee to dump me.

I had made a reservation so we got seated right away. We agreed that we probably had crossed paths before. We lived only a couple of miles from each other. We shopped at the same super-market and nearby mall. For years we both took the same train downtown from the Palatine station. We frequented the same local bar and restaurant called Brandt's.

Marilee was a recent widow who had been married to her husband for forty-four years. He was very ill for the last five years of his life. He cried a lot and felt helpless as she took him all over looking for an accurate diagnosis. He made several ambulance rides to the local hospital because he became unconscious and could not breathe. Each time they were able to bring him back.

Marilee took him to Rush and Northwestern—both teaching hospitals in Chicago. But neither of the teaching hospitals got his diagnosis right. They went to Mayo Clinic and liked the care there, but they still didn't find out exactly what Bob had. Finally Marilee took him to UCLA Medical Center in Los Angeles where Bob received an accurate diagnosis.

He had hydrocephalus which is a form of water on the brain. It affected him profoundly. He had great difficulty walking and talking. He could not dress himself. His memory failed him. He was delusional. He urinated in his pants. He hated living with the terrible symptoms and was angry with Marilee for calling ambulances and having the hospital save his life when he would stop breathing and become unconscious. He told her over and over not to call an ambulance again. He kept saying he would rather die than live with the crippling symptoms of hydrocephalus. Finally, one day when he had a severe attack, he refused medical care. He passed away at home within an hour.

Marilee lived with her family until she married Bob when she turned twenty-one. She had never lived alone. She slept with her mother or older sister before she moved out and married Bob. She had never slept alone. Now she was all alone and afraid of the night.

She would lie in bed fully awake terrified that someone would break in and do her harm. She longed for male companionship and took to the internet to find someone to love. By the time I met her she had been on a few dates but the men she liked didn't seem to be interested in her. They never called her back. I certainly knew what she was talking about.

So far each of our recent efforts to find someone special online had failed, and we both arrived really hoping that this night would be different.

I didn't mention my bipolar illness until our third date. Marilee was a trained psychiatric nurse and noticed what she thought could be minor symptoms of a psychiatric disorder. So she wasn't really too surprised when I told her about my illness.

I spoke about all of the medications, the long hospitalizations, and the 200 electric shock treatments. Instead of seeing me as a sick, perhaps dangerous individual, she saw me as a rare, courageous person who defied nearly impossible odds of overcoming a severe mental illness.

In her years as a psychiatric nurse she had not seen even one patient recover as well as me. Instead of being afraid of me she was drawn to me. I couldn't believe my luck. Marilee was kind and smart, very attractive and sexy, and she viewed my history with severe bipolar disorder as a very positive attribute. Best of all she really liked me.

At first I didn't really trust my newfound good fortune, and I was afraid of saying or doing something that would ruin it. I was especially afraid of intimacy. Perhaps because I am bipolar I had a sad history of failed intimate relationships.

Marilee had her reservations too. She had been with the same man for forty-four years and loved him deeply. Was there room in her heart for someone else so soon?

She wasn't really sure what she was looking for so she decided she would be safer having only a summer romance with me.

I continued to see Dr. Francis every Tuesday at 1:30 p.m. I saw Dr. Easton every month and always took my medications as prescribed.

I had a hard time believing it, but I seemed to be having some real stability in my life. Both doctors told me it would be hard for anyone to tell I was bipolar unless I told them about it.

My recovery was so slow I hardly noticed it, but others who knew me when I was very ill were pleasantly surprised at my progress. When I walked I still moved slowly, but the lurching from side to side had stopped. I was better at looking people in the eye. Best of all the strong suicidal urges seemed to be asleep.

Marilee and I both loved movies and often saw a movie before we went out for dinner. I didn't have a lot of money and told

224 | THOMAS RICKE

Marilee I couldn't really afford go to dinner more than once a week, so she would invite me over for a home-cooked meal.

Every so often the electricity in my apartment building failed and left me with candles in the dark, no hot water, no television, no stove, and no air conditioning.

After a couple of months of dating Marilee, the power in my apartment went out again. Con Ed said it was caused by a serious problem in a substation that might take days to fix.

It was in the beginning of summer. I told Marilee that my life was becoming totally dark and hot. I couldn't take a shower or even cook a meal in the microwave. There was no hot water, and I needed candles and a flashlight to walk around after dark.

She thought about it for a few moments and then invited Lucky and me to stay at her house until the electricity found its way back to my apartment.

When we arrived Lucky was afraid of Marilee and hid safely behind my legs. It was a wonderful three or four days for all of us. Our intimacy was a healthy mix of mutual affection and excitement. Those few days marked the very fragile beginning of a new and hopeful chapter in my life.

When they were healthy, my parents would spend at least six months of every year visiting their five children. We lived all over the place. Sue lived near Toronto, Kathy in Traverse City, Peggy in Sacramento, Bernie in a Detroit suburb, and me in New York City and then the Chicago area.

My father loved to drive so my parents would literally drive from coast to coast and north to Traverse City, Michigan, and Toronto. They would spend at least two or three weeks at each of our homes.

There came a time when my father's age wouldn't let him drive safely for long distances. So my parents would fly to Bernie's house and we would all visit them there. Eventually we started a tradition that we would visit my parents at Bernie's house during the Fourth of July holiday. My parents would stay with Bernie, and the rest of us would stay at local hotels.

After both my parents passed away we continued the Fourth of

July tradition as an annual family reunion at Bernie's house. We called it "Ricke fest."

There was a reunion two and a half months after Marilee and I met. We went together. I wanted Marie and my brother and sisters to meet Marilee so they would know I was in what seemed like a healthy relationship.

After the last years with Maura, the weird relationship with Margaret and the totally failed marriage to Barbara, my family viewed my history with women the same as Dr. Easton when he told me, "You really know how to pick them, Tom."

I was introducing Marilee to my family when Sue's husband Karl walked over to meet us. He had a great sense of humor and was always quick with a joke. I told him Marilee was a psychiatric nurse whom Medicare paid to take care of me because her services were less expensive than hospitalization.

At first he seemed to believe me and didn't know what to say. My sister Kathy was nearby and heard me. When she broke out in laughter, Karl caught on.

Before I became so ill I had a pretty good sense of humor, but it disappeared when manic depression claimed me. This was probably the first joke I tried to tell in a decade or more. It sure was fun.

Chapter 20

After Ricke fest that year Marilee and I started to live together part-time. I would come with Lucky after I got off work on Thursday evenings and stay until Monday morning when Marilee left for work. The only days we didn't see each other were Tuesdays and Wednesdays. Sometimes we would email each other on those days.

Apparently I was the first one to use the L word. Marilee remembers I wrote that I loved her in an email. After that we told each other we were in love quite often. After all those years of profound sorrow I was actually happy. I was in a loving, stable relationship, and no one could tell I was mentally ill.

Both of Marilee's children, Lisa and David, lived only twenty minutes away, and we would get together with them and their children quite frequently. They thought I was somewhat distant, quiet, and shy, but they never even suspected I was bipolar.

Marilee had a terrific relationship with her two children and five grandchildren. So we see them often. In comparison, I see Marie and her family only two or three times a year.

After a few months Marilee's five grandchildren began to call me "Grandpa Tom." During that year's Christmas holidays

Marilee and I decided to live together full-time when my lease expired in April, which happened to be about a year after we met.

Marilee told her children that we planned to live together at a holiday gathering at Lisa's house. After they heard the news, they were worried about their mother. They knew me for about eight months, but they wondered if they really knew me well.

Was Marilee too vulnerable since their father died? Did she realize what she was getting into? How would I treat her when we lived under the same roof? Did they really know me? Was I trustworthy? Was I really a good man?

David decided he would call his mother and try to talk her out of living with me. I had some difficulty getting my passport renewed, and David asked his mother, "What kind of a person has trouble getting a passport?"

She told him she was "very fond" of me, and losing me would be much too traumatic for her. She didn't want to be without me in her life. After that conversation I became an accepted member of the family.

Whatever the surgeon did in my first back surgery stopped working and I found myself with more back pain than ever. It was a screaming pain that kept me from sleeping. The pills helped some, but even the strongest pain meds didn't end the suffering.

I had to use a wheelchair to manage any distances. In our house we put chairs in a line every twenty feet or so, and I would hobble from chair to chair. Sitting down gave some relief.

When she was nineteen Marie had major back surgery. I needed the same type of operation. The surgeon would fuse the vertebrae in the bottom third of my spine using four rods and eight screws and some cadaver bone. I had confidence in the surgeon, and the pain was so bad I welcomed the surgery.

I was already living with Marilee at the time. She took me to the hospital and waited patiently for the results of the seven-hour surgery. I woke up in a hospital bed in a private room. I was on oxygen and had I.V.s in my arm. I began to hallucinate as a side effect of the anesthesia. I saw men dressed in black suits and carrying guns come into the room to shoot me. They were mafia gangsters from Miami. I had to get away from them. I rolled off of the bed onto the floor tearing an I.V. from my arm and the oxygen from my nose. A loud alarm sounded and nurses rushed in to help me back in bed and reattach the I.V.

After a few days they transferred me to a rehab facility that was attached to the main hospital. The rooms there were the same as hospital rooms. I was to stay for at least two weeks to practice walking a few steps at a time and climbing up stairs. Marilee came to visit every single day.

During the second week of my stay there she brought me the obituary section of the local newspaper. The first obit was for Barbara Saccameno, my ex-wife's maiden name. Barb's breast cancer from many years ago had returned to claim her life. After our toxic three-year marriage I think we both felt some relief that it was over. But not this. She was supposed to start over and find happiness in her life after Tom.

I felt sorry for her children. They were much too young to lose their mother. Despite her personality problems, Barb had been a good mother.

I was stuck in the rehab unable to visit the funeral home or attend her final service. The last time we met was in court. After the divorce we each had agreed to pay half of our debt. I was to pay our $35,000 Mastercard bill, and she was to pay somewhat less that was due on the second mortgage that was still in my name.

She hadn't paid a dime on what was left on the second mortgage, and I was being harassed day and night by bill collectors.

My credit was ruined. So I sued her over her failure to pay anything toward her part of our debt. When we got to court she promised the judge she would start making payments, but she never did. I eventually dropped the lawsuit.

If I was the devil when we divorced, I can only imagine what she told her children, relatives, and friends about me when I sued her. Perhaps it was for the best that I couldn't attend her services. I might not have been welcome.

When I left the rehab and finally returned home, I was still walking very slowly and unsteadily. I couldn't drive right away. A physical therapist came to the house every day for three weeks. Then I continued physical therapy for two hours a day three days a week at a nearby facility. I made progress with walking very slowly, but I feared I'd never walk normally. I walked slowly before my back surgeries, and I still walk slowly today.

Every few yards Marilee has to wait for a moment for me to catch up. This walking difficulty is a direct side effect of the medicine I take so it probably will be with me for the rest of my life.

Nine months after my major back surgery my back started to hurt again, hurt as badly as before the operation. I was despondent.

I never even thought the surgery wouldn't work. What was I going to do now? What would happen if my bipolar illness awakened? Would I have to live the rest of my life in a wheelchair on pain meds in addition to all the psychiatric medicine I have to take? How would the back torture affect my manic depression?

The MRI showed vertebrae pinching nerves again. The vertebra on top of the fusion was rubbing against the vertebra directly on top of it. The surgeon told me I would need a third back surgery to fix the painful problem. He would have to insert what they called a "cage" in between the affected vertebrae so they could not pinch nerves. When I asked the surgeon what could I do if the third surgery didn't work, he told me he wouldn't let that happen. So far so good. It's been five years since that surgery and the most I have experienced is an occasional stiff back.

After I recovered from the last surgery my middle sister, Kathy, had an unusual session with her dentist. She went to him for what she thought was a tooth abscess.

After his examination the dentist told Kathy it looked like she had a tumor in her mouth, and she should go to her regular doctor for treatment.

She was an excellent freelance writer for the *Detroit Free Press*. She lived in Traverse City, Michigan.

Occasionally Kathy covered news stories from her area of the state, but she wrote mostly feature stories that earned prominent placement in the newspaper's Sunday feature section or Sunday magazine.

Her husband Bob Prentice had trained to be a speech therapist but worked at a really good but expensive local private school instead because the job provided free tuition for their daughters Kaitlin and Lilly.

Traverse City is a great summer town on the shores of Lake Michigan. Marie spent some summers there with her cousins. She was very close to Kathy.

The *Detroit Free Press* suffered a long strike. One of the unions, the Newspaper Guild, represented the paper's editorial staff. The paper's top editors were not in the union. Kathy wasn't a union member because she was a freelance writer, not an employee.

A few reporters broke with the union and helped the paper continue to publish, but most of them stayed out.

The editors still working at the paper put a lot of pressure on Kathy to try to get her to cross the picket line and be a reporter for the strike edition of the paper. Kathy refused, and when the strike was over months later the editors told her she could not work for the paper any longer. They were obviously punishing her for her refusal to work during the strike.

Kathy eventually found work writing for a news outlet on the internet.

Kathy's tumor was malignant and the cancer had spread to her throat. Worse, the chemotherapy didn't seem to be working for her. She joined an experimental program offered by the University of Michigan's hospital.

She tried very hard to be optimistic, but it wasn't easy.

When I talked to her I didn't know what to say so I wrote her this email:

"First, there is always hope. We all know stories of cancer patients who live far beyond their doctor's prediction. Marilee's good friend Joan has breast cancer. She was given a year to live a dozen years ago and she is still with us.

"There were times when I wanted to die more than I wanted to live. I have had three very close suicide attempts. Twice I was in a coma. After I recovered from the bipolar madness I would ask myself why I was still here, what difference has my life made to anyone.

"Your answer to that question is that you've made a huge positive difference in the lives you have touched.

"You raised two wonderful young women who face their lives armed with your example of constructive curiosity and heart-warming affection.

"They have learned from you that it is very important to succeed in careers that reward with self-esteem and self-confidence. They have also learned from you how it is even more important to cultivate friendships with love and respect.

"Your relationship with Bob gives us all a powerful example of how a good marriage can truly benefit both partners. You have had the same close friends for decades. They are all better off with you in their lives.

"Then there is your writing. You have the gift of touching your readers with words that make them stop and think about what really matters in their lives.

"When others gave up hope that I could recover from the powerful mental illness that ruined many years of my life you stuck by me and that helped me in my recovery.

"What I am trying to say is that you have made a very positive difference in the lives of everyone who has been fortunate enough to know you and be loved by you.

"As Robert Frost wrote, 'I took the road less traveled and that made all the difference.' May you keep leading us down that road for years to come."

Kathy told me she really appreciated the email, but she was not going to indulge in "wishful thinking" anymore. She had been asked to leave the experimental cancer-fighting program because it just wasn't working for her. There were absolutely no positive results. All she could do now was to prepare for the end. Her last words to me were over the phone. "Tom, I love you."

Then she hung up.

Kathy died at home with her children and husband at her side. She had made arrangements to donate her body to science. What was left would be cremated. She didn't want any funeral ceremony. She didn't want to burden her family and friends.

Despite her wishes our family decided to hold a reception for her memory. Many family members, neighbors, and friends crowded into a fairly large room.

She loved to make quilts so her family hung some of them high on the walls. They also posted many family pictures lower on the walls.

There were two tables covered with her writings for the *Detroit Free Press*.

One article really stunned us. It was a first-hand account of her surviving a major heart attack. None of us outside of her husband and children knew she suffered the attack. Kathy didn't want to burden us with her problems.

After the string quartet stopped playing and most of the guests had left, Kaitlin and Lilly ran into a very cold Lake Michigan with their clothes on. Their mother probably would have joined them.

On the way home I was thinking that with Kathy's and my parents' deaths. The Ricke family had shrunk from seven to four in the last couple of years. I was the oldest, and I would soon find out I had serious medical conditions that had nothing to do with my mental illness or my back.

I was hospitalized three times in Good Shepherd Hospital while I worked there for coughing up and vomiting blood. I received three separate diagnoses, one with each admission. None of them determined the real cause of the bleeding.

During one admission a doctor made a big deal out of my bipolar illness accusing me of making up the bleeding issue.

I finally visited a well-known specialist who lowered the dose of blood thinner I was talking every day. I had been taking Coumadin since I had blood clots during the late nineties.

The unwanted bleeding stopped when the dosage was lowered.

I developed a rather serious case of COPD, a result of my

childhood asthma and smoking. I had quit smoking years ago right after I left Barbara, but apparently the damage had already been done.

I have been hospitalized six times in the past three years for severe pneumonia. In each of these incidents I was starved for oxygen. It scared the hell out of me.

No matter how hard I tried I couldn't breathe. My lungs would not expand to take in air. I struggled. I inhaled as hard as I could, but the air would not go down into my lungs. I could not move. While I waited for the ambulance and its oxygen, I felt my life slipping away.

During one of the more recent hospitalizations they had to put me on intubation—a machine they put down your throat that breathes for you.

After the drug that made me sleep through the intubation wore off a doctor in the intensive care unit told me that I came very close to dying during the ordeal.

During each of those hospitalizations they gave me oxygen and I.V. antibiotics during a four- to five-day stay. I have already been hospitalized twice this year for pneumonia. Despite many tests doctors have been unable to determine exactly what is causing my severe breathing issues.

Marilee visited me every day I was in the hospital for my back surgeries and my inability to breathe. My breathing illness was exceptionally hard for her because it was a vivid remainder of her husband's bad health before he died.

Her Bob had difficulty breathing as one of his symptoms. Marilee had to call an ambulance for him several times. One time she would never forget happened on a Christmas Eve when Bob was intubated before going to intensive care.

The time I was put on intubation was also on a Christmas Eve.

The same ambulance and crew that serviced Bob took me to Northwestern Community Hospital, the same hospital that took care of Bob before he died.

As Marilee drove to the hospital that night she couldn't stop the vivid, painful memories of her taking care of her husband.

Would it be the same with me?

In previous years when I would see a man or woman walking around pulling a green oxygen tank hooked up to their nose I would wince and think, "Thank God that could never happen to me."

After my last hospitalization I was given oxygen equipment that I am supposed to use when I get too short of breath.

I have a large unit next to the TV in the family room, which I use when I am home. I have a portable unit that I carry over my shoulder when I am walking around. I use this sometimes when I am out and about.

During my last visit to my lung doctor he told me that my lung capacity was only forty percent, and it would probably never get better.

Thank you, Marlboro Lights. I knew smoking was not good for me, but I certainly didn't think I would suffer so much so many years after I had quit.

On our most recent visit to the Dominican Republic I had to take my oxygen with me and use it at Chicago's O'Hare Airport where you have to walk for what seems like miles. Today I become short of breath, but I am not bad enough to need the oxygen.

Marie quit her job as a speech therapist for small children when she was pregnant with her first child. After she had Eve she and Jim bought a house. They had another girl they named Isabel after they moved into their new home. Right now Eve is six and Isabel is two.

Before Isabel came along Marie spent every waking hour playing with and reading to Eve. Her constant attention paid off.

Eve just started kindergarten and she can already read at a third-grade level. I think she is very smart for her age, but I also think all those hours and days Marie spent reading the same children's books over and over have a lot to do with Eve's ability to read so well at her age.

Jim has a monster commute. It takes him about two hours each way. He has to get up and catch a bus to the train before his children wake up. By the time he gets home they are usually sound asleep for the night.

He did get permission to work at home for one or two days each week, but he often has to go to the office on those days so he can attend necessary meetings and do things you just can't do at home.

Chapter 21

I have been seeing Dr. Francis every Tuesday for nearly thirty years. In her opinion I have not lived a normal adult life, not until fairly recently. During my decades of professional achievement she thinks I was most likely hypomanic much of the time. The milder form of mania fueled my success with increased creativity, energy, euphoria, and desire and drive for professional success. It gave me a rather charismatic personality. I could be the life of the party and the voice of success to follow in business meetings.

I hate to think that any professional or personal success I attained was due to the symptoms of a mental illness, but the facts show my life as a series of dramatic ups and downs, totally consistent with the symptoms of my rapid cycling bipolar disorder.

On the upside there was a life of professional success in the media, politics, and corporate America that was not "normal," according to Dr. Francis. She says flying on corporate jets or attending state dinners or visiting the President in the White House would not be normal activities for most people.

People who consider themselves normal usually don't end up as senior vice presidents of major American companies. They don't become chief speechwriters for the governor of New York at age twenty-seven.

There's a symptom of manic depression that people don't talk about much. I would call it an insatiable sexual and emotional appetite. No matter how much affection and sex there is in a relationship, it's never enough if you are bipolar. At least that was my experience. Once I was properly medicated the promiscuous behavior just stopped.

Then there's the other side of manic depression. Sure, there are the normal periods of depression from life experiences—the untimely deaths of loved ones, the loss of a job or best friend or a terrible loneliness. These and other events will cause normal people to suffer from some depression, but the mad sadness of manic depression is much worse. It is more intense, more painful, and it lasts a lot longer.

Bipolar depression can be triggered by sad events in a person's life, but then it takes on a life of its own. This is what happened to me after I lost my job at Kraft Foods. Every thought, every sound, every movement, every breath seemed to cause unbearable psychic pain.

Ending that pain can become a person's fondest wish. If only there was a switch to press to make it go away. Suicide can become that switch. Ending one's life will surely end one's pain. That's why as many as seventy percent of people with untreated bipolar disorder attempt suicide. That's why twenty percent of people with untreated manic depression die from suicide. I believe that the vast majority of people who kill themselves or attempt to kill themselves suffer from mental illness. I certainly did.

Somehow I survived three serious attempts. I don't know why I lived and my son died. I really wanted to die. I felt I had to die. If I owned a gun, I would have been dead years ago. I wanted to drift off to sleep and never wake up. Twice I ended up in a coma. I am told I came as close to dying as you can get without dying.

Yes, I had three attempts when my life was saved in the emergency room, but suicide haunted me day and night in between those attempts. I thought about it frequently. Sometimes it would come to me when there was no immediate reason for wanting my death, when I just thought it would be nice to die.

The powerful sexual urges, the dramatic ups and the frightening downs, the suicidal ideation, the absence of any stability—all this and more made it very difficult for me to have good, mutually rewarding relationships.

Today I consider myself a very fortunate man.

The voices of suicide have been largely quiet for the past ten years. I think about it from time to time, but the thoughts are usually brief and quiet memories of the painful past. They are not powerful urges to do it. They are polite and civil, almost like a college lecture.

I still see Dr. Francis every week and Dr. Easton every couple of months. They both say I am stable now, more stable than any other time since they have known me.

I am not full of myself as I was when I became manic. I am not depressed. I am certainly not suicidal. I am not flying high in corporate jets or being saved in hospital emergency rooms. I am leading a fairly normal life.

How did this happen? How did I defy all the odds to find a rather normal life? For the past thirty years I have taken every pill that was prescribed by Dr. Easton. I endured every electric shock treatment. I saw Dr. Francis every week for nearly thirty years and Dr. Easton on a regular basis for the same amount of time. No matter what, I always did what I was told to do even if I hated it. I was totally compliant.

I improved inch by inch, so slowly I hardly noticed it. Slow but steady. It took many years to get to where I am today.

If you or a loved one is suffering from mental illness I would like you to do what I did. Find a good doctor and/or therapist and follow their every suggestion. Trust them. I was very fortunate to have excellent doctors caring for me. There are good doctors out there.

The best way to find them is referrals from satisfied patients. They tell me my recovery is rare. They tell me it is nearly impossible to live a normal life after being as sick as I was from mental illness. As doctor Easton said, "You are sick as you can be from mental illness."

Yet, here I am finishing a book. Here I am actually happy most of the time. My story proves that it is possible to lead a normal life after severe mental illness.

My relationship with Marilee is the foundation of my stability. We've been together eight years now. We are not legally married, but we introduce each other as "my husband" or "my wife." We rarely argue, and when we do, we don't keep it going. We always end it as soon as we can, and we always make up right away.

We have a lot in common. We both love going to the movies. We both love music. She loved classical and never bothered with rock and roll or the blues or any other kind of music. Now that she has listened to my music she really likes the Beatles and the Rolling Stones, and I am learning to like classical music.

We are both affectionate. We both love to be intimate, not as much as in our earlier years, but not bad for our seventies.

We plan to be at each other's side until the end.

Thanksgiving at Marie's is still a family tradition. We all come for the annual dinner. Marilee and I always come. Maura always is there. She used to bring her husband Jerry, but now she comes alone since he died. Of course Jim and Marie and Isabel and Eve are there. Jim's mom used to come, but she won't be there this year. The drive from Alabama is difficult for her.

This is the picture I want to make at the end of this book. Thanksgiving at Marie's. Marilee and Maura becoming good friends. Maura and I being friends. Each of us trying to remember the best of our past while teasing each other in a friendly way. Marie is so happy that her parents are getting along so well.

This is my life now. Normal, stable, full of mutual love and affection, actually loving my life, loving being alive. I am so lucky to be alive.

Chances are I will be like this for the rest of my life, but it is not 100 percent certain. As Dr. Easton once told me, "The only thing you can say for sure about manic depression is that it is totally unpredictable."

ABOUT THE AUTHOR

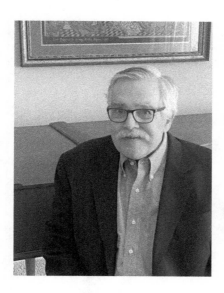

Thomas Ricke's writing skills were the foundation of his success in the media, politics and corporate communications. He was a staff writer for the Detroit Free Press and an editorial writer for the New York Daily News. He wrote speeches for the Governor of New York State, the Mayor of New York City and the publisher of Black Enterprise Magazine. He worked in corporate America where he became a senior vice president of Kraft Foods. Symptoms of his severe manic depression caused him to lose his position at Kraft. He lost everything of value in his life. His 16-year-old son, who was also bipolar, committed suicide. His wife of 22 years divorced him. He was never able to work at a full-time job again, but he never gave up. Today Mr. Ricke is living a normal retirement life in the Chicago area with his significant other, Marilee. His suicidal madness has been silent for many years. Mr. Ricke is available for speeches and interviews.